How Fat Works

PHILIP A. WOOD

How Fat Works

Harvard University Press
Cambridge, Massachusetts
London, England
2006

Library of Congress Cataloging-in-Publication Data

Wood, Philip A.
  How fat works / Philip A. Wood.
    p. ; cm.
  Includes bibliographical references and index.
  ISBN 0-674-01947-4 (alk. paper)
    1. Lipids.   2. Lipids—Metabolism.   3. Adipose tissues—Metabolism.
  4. Obesity—Genetic aspects.   5. Obesity—Prevention.   I. Title.
    [DNLM: 1. Lipids—metabolism.   2. Adipose Tissues—metabolism.
  3. Obesity—genetics.   4. Obesity—prevention and control. QU 85 W878h 2006]
  QP751.W66 2006
  612.3'97—dc22   2005051357

In memory of my early mentors,
Thomas E. Chapman and Joseph E. Smith

Contents

Acknowledgments

I am very grateful to the many people who helped make possible the creation of this book. First, I thank my editor at Harvard University Press, Ann Downer-Hazell, who saw the potential for this project when many others did not. She helped in many ways to craft this book into one with a mission: to bridge basic science with clinical disease issues. Many thanks go to a group I meet with weekly known affectionately as "Lipid Breakfast." The idea for the book and many of the topics covered were spawned from discussions with this group. Of this group, I am indebted to Albert Oberman, Vera Bittner, Carroll Harmon, William Bradley, James Shikany, and Jere Segrest, who all read chapters, answered many questions, and supplied helpful feedback. I especially acknowledge the efforts of Frank Franklin, also of that group, who read the entire manuscript and offered many helpful suggestions and was a continuous source of information and encouragement. I want to thank, too, Barbara Gower, Tim Nagy, Kevin Pawlik, Lisa Guay-Woodford, and Bob Kesterson, who also read chapters and provided helpful comments. Lee Griner edited early versions of the book and very importantly contributed to making an early draft readable for consideration by others. David Fisher produced the graphics, always with ready willingness to keep making a few more changes. Many thanks to Kate Schmit for her outstanding contribution on the final copy editing.

I also thank my family for their continued support. My wife, Judy, was always there with encouragement and many helpful ideas, and she read multiple versions of the manuscript. I am especially blessed in having Judy—along with our two sons, John and Joseph—making my life rich and full. I am grateful to my parents, Donna and William Wood, for a lifetime of support and encouragement. I also thank my mentors in the field of of metabolism and genetics, Henry Baker, Arthur Beaudet, and William O'Brien. Finally, I dedicate this book to the memory of Thomas Chapman and Joseph Smith. These two highly regarded professors and mentors made lasting contributions to my career development and my interest in metabolic disease.

Abbreviations

ACC	acetyl-CoA carboxylase
AgRP	agouti-related protein
ATP	adenosine triphosphate
BMI	body mass index
CART	cocaine and amphetamine regulated transcript
CCK	cholecystokinin
CoA	coenzyme A
CPT	carnitine palmitoyltransferase
DHA	docosahexaenoic acid
DM	diabetes mellitus
DRV	Daily reference values
%DV	%Daily Values
EPA	eicosapentaenoic acid
ETF	electron transport flavoprotein
FDA	Food and Drug Administration
FFM	fat free mass
FH	familial hypercholesterolemia
GI	glycemic index
GLP-1	glucagon-like peptide 1
HDL	high-density lipoprotein
HELLP	hypertension, elevated liver enzymes, and low platelets
HMG-CoA	3-hydroxy-3-methyl-glutaryl-CoA
IDL	intermediate-density lipoprotein
IMCL	intramyocellular lipid
IRS	insulin receptor substrate

LCAD	long-chain acyl-CoA dehydrogenase
LCHAD	long-chain hydroxyacyl-CoA dehydrogenase
LDL	low-density lipoprotein
MC-4	melanocortin-4
MCAD	medium-chain acyl-CoA dehydrogenase
M/SCHAD	medium/short-chain hydroxyacyl-CoA dehydrogenase
MUFA	monounsaturated fatty acid
NAD$^+$	nicotinamide adenine dinucleotide
NADP$^+$	nicotinamide adenine dinucleotide phosphate
NAFLD	nonalcoholic fatty liver disease
NASH	nonalcoholic steatohepatitis
NLEA	Nutrition Labeling and Education Act
NPY	neuropeptide Y
PI3	phosphatidylinositol-3
PKU	phenylketonuria
POMC	pro-opiomelanocortin
PP	peroxisomal proliferator
PPAR	peroxisomal proliferator-activated receptor
PUFA	polyunsaturated fatty acid
REE	resting energy expenditure
RMR	resting metabolic rate
SCAD	short-chain acyl-CoA dehydrogenase
SIDS	sudden infant death syndrome
SNP	single nucleotide polymorphism
SREBP	sterol-response element binding protein
TZD	thiazolidinedione
VLCAD	very long-chain acyl-CoA dehydrogenase
VLDL	very low-density lipoprotein

How Fat Works

Introduction: Lessons from a Mouse

For many years I have been fascinated by metabolism and the genes, nutrients, and drugs that influence it. Given the growing epidemic of obesity, diabetes, and related diseases, more and more people are beginning to share that interest. I wrote this book to help students and healthcare professionals, as well as the general reader, understand more fully the processes of fat metabolism and the diseases of excess fat.

Much of my research has been done using mice that have been genetically modified to alter their fat metabolism. Since the mid-1980s, my research group has developed "gene knockout" mouse models to ask the question, "What happens if a body cannot complete the process of fat burning?" By studying mice with different genetic mutations that interfere with fat burning (fatty acid oxidation), we have investigated important mechanistic components of the common diseases of fat metabolism described in this book. (Mouse models are discussed more fully in Schuler and Wood, 2002.) Our experiments explore the complex interaction of genetics, nutrition, and drugs on fat metabolism and related diseases.

Major concepts of the molecular basis of obesity were learned from the mutant mouse known as *obese*. This mouse model has led the way to a whole new understanding of obesity. In elegant experiments done in the 1960s at the Jackson Laboratory in Bar Harbor, Maine, Douglas Coleman showed that this severely obese mouse was deficient in a blood-borne factor that regulates appetite and activity level (Coleman 1978). This factor apparently prevents development of obesity in a normal mouse. In 1994, Jeffrey Friedman and colleagues at Rockefeller University discovered and cloned the gene underlying this disease and identified this critical factor, a hormone they called *leptin* (Zhang et al. 1994). This genetic approach revealed leptin deficiency as the cause of extreme obesity in the mouse. Eventually a few human patients were found with the same genetic deficiency. Although the inherited human disease is extremely rare, the discovery of its mechanism offered new insight.

From these important lessons, scientists learned that body fat *(adipose tissue)* does much more than "just" store fat molecules. Adipose cells *(adipocytes)* secrete essential hormones, such as leptin, and other important molecules that interact with the organs of the body, such as the brain. These signals are involved with appetite control, activity level, and regulation of metabolic rate.

Other mouse mutants have revealed many essential components for maintaining a lean and healthy state. Multiple genes affect regulation of fat synthesis and fat oxidation, which must be kept in balance (Wood 2004). When there is too much of the former and not enough of the latter, excess fat builds up and may lead not only to obesity but to other serious problems, such as insulin resistance and diabetes. Thus, mouse models that develop obesity, insulin resistance, and diabetes—or in contrast are genetically resistant to these diseases—have contributed enormously to our understanding of the primary genetics of fat metabolism and various aspects of diseases of excess fat.

From the genetics of these processes of metabolism, scientists are learning the important "pivot points" that are often influenced by nutrients and drugs. For example, scientists may know the DNA sequence of a particular gene encoding an enzyme involved with fat oxidation. That gene sequence information is important, but it is only part of the story. The expression of the enzyme gene (the process of synthesizing the enzyme) may be turned "up or down" by a regulatory protein encoded by a different gene. The regulatory protein may be drastically affected by the presence or absence of a particular nutrient—e.g., a specific fatty acid—or a drug. As you can see, the sequence of steps and signals becomes complicated very quickly.

My goal in this book is to explain the influences of genetics, nutrition, exercise, and drugs on the storage and burning of body fat. The topic also requires explanations of what I call the diseases and syndromes of excess fat: obesity, insulin resistance, metabolic syndrome, type 2 diabetes, and related disease processes of high concentrations of cholesterol and triglycerides in the blood. The main focus of this book is both the normal physiology and the pathophysiology of fat metabolism. It is offered as a book grounded in basic science but with discussions of clinical diseases offered to enliven what is too often perceived as tedious biochemistry with no practical relevance. I have also included some observations about related issues, such as nutrient labeling on packaged foods, alternative medicine and diets, clinical trials, and media coverage of health research.

Instruction for clinical care of patients with these disorders is beyond the scope of this book. My target audience includes medical, nursing, nutrition, and graduate students in their basic science years. I also expect that practicing healthcare professionals wanting a basic science refresher—as well as the ambitious general reader interested in a deeper understanding of the topic—will find the book useful. Scientists have learned much from mouse models about the diseases of excess fat, and we must now apply this information to the very serious health problems affecting so many people today.

PART I

Problems of Excess Fat and Cholesterol

CHAPTER 1

The Burden of Obesity

Many believe there is an epidemic of obesity in the United States. Obesity, much more than a cosmetic problem, is perhaps the most conspicuous reason to understand how fat works. Obesity is strongly associated with many serious diseases or syndromes, such as metabolic syndrome, diabetes, hypertension, and arthritis. This chapter describes the different types of body fat, or adipose tissue, and how they function in different locations in the body. Adipose tissue is an important organ of the body; it functions not only as a "sink" for fatty acids but also as a hormone-secreting organ. One such hormone, leptin, has direct effects on the brain and fat metabolism. Surprisingly, individuals who have too little body fat are at risk for some of the same diseases, such as insulin resistance and diabetes, that commonly occur among obese persons.

Much of what we know of fat metabolism comes from the study of genetic disorders of obesity. Scientists have learned about the normal processes of appetite control, feeding behavior, and hormones derived from adipose tissue through these studies.

Obesity Is a Health Risk

I begin with obesity because it is the most evident reason for investigating how excess fat affects health and disease. Defined as the disease of having excess body fat (a more precise definition may be found in Chapter 2), obesity is in the news almost daily because many people, but not all, believe an epidemic of obesity is occurring in the United States today (Wickelgren 1998). An economist at RAND recently showed that obesity was more costly than smoking and alcohol abuse (Sturm 2002). In general terms, he said that obesity increases risks of disease as much as 20 years of aging does. Almost a quarter of the people in the United States are now obese, and another 55% are overweight. Also, obesity in children is at an all-time high (Rocchini 2002). The National Longitudinal Survey of Youth reports that between 1986 and 1998, the prevalence of overweight has increased 21.5% among non-Hispanic black children, 21.8% among Hispanic children, and 12.3% among non-Hispanic white children (Strauss and Pollack 2001). Obesity is an extremely important risk factor in the development of metabolic syndrome, previously known as syndrome X (Chapter 5), and the accompanying problems of insulin resistance, hypertension, blood coagulation problems, and cardiovascular disease. Of course these problems can lead to the real biggies, type 2 diabetes and heart attacks. The Centers for Disease Control and Prevention (CDC) does not have complete data as yet; however, clinically the incidence of type 2 diabetes in children and adolescents is increasing at an alarming rate (Rosenbloom et al. 1999). No ethnic group is free of diabetes in children, but the disease affects disproportionately more American Indian, Mexican American, African American, and Pacific Islander youth. In Pima Indians of Arizona, the 15–19-year-old age group has a prevalence of type 2 diabetes of 5%. In clinic-based studies of children newly diagnosed with diabetes, the percentage of those with type 2 has increased from <5% in 1994 to >30–50% in subsequent years (National Diabetes Education Program 2004). This means that in less than a decade, the predominant form of diabetes in children has shifted from type 1 (insulin dependent) to type 2 diabetes, which is often associated with obesity.

Obesity Occurs When Calorie Intake Exceeds Output

While the social, personal, and political causes of obesity are complex and intractable, at the level of the individual's metabolism obesity is not mysterious. Many people do not have an activity level high enough to offset the amount of calories they take in (Pi-Sunyer 2003). The disease may be more complex, however, involving an individual's inherited characteristics in basal metabolism and fat storage, in brain regulation of feeding patterns and exercise, and a host of unknown factors. Yes, some people have genetically determined factors that overwhelmingly influence their propensity to store extra fat or their feelings of hunger versus satiety (Comuzzie and Allison 1998). These extremely rare patients will have a difficult time with weight control. In most people, genetic effects are subtler and can often be overcome by behavioral changes. An obese patient will lose body fat if forcefully restricted to a reduced-calorie intake matched by exercise-induced calorie expenditure. Obesity is curable.

We know this because gastric bypass surgery, in which the stomach is drastically reduced in size (to 30–60 ml) and is disconnected from the upper small intestine (duodenum) and reconnected to the middle small intestine (jejunum), will markedly reduce the patient's body fat and often cure insulin resistance. This surgery is reserved for morbidly obese people who have a body mass index (BMI) greater than 40 or those with BMI over 35 with other risk factors for severe disease like diabetes, hypertension, or cardiovascular disease. I will explain more about BMI in Chapter 2. Obesity is a behavioral, psychological, genetic, nutritional, and metabolic disease. Its treatment is complicated by many things—including a cultural propensity to see obesity as a moral failing and a toxic fast-food culture that encourages sedentary lifestyles.

The pathogenesis of obesity has several components (Campfield, Smith, and Burn 1998). Inherited causes of obesity often result from genetic changes that influence feeding behavior and metabolic characteristics. There are also many social implications of obesity. Unfortunately, obese people are often depicted as being weak-willed. Some obese patients, however, are able to change their way of thinking about how they're going to deal with life and how they want to look and feel. They may have inherited characteristics that predispose them to obesity, but they can and do help themselves, some with the aid of drug therapy or gastric bypass surgery. Unfortunately, many will cycle repeatedly through weight loss and weight gain—what has been called the "rhythm method of girth control."

Many people overeat when they are stressed or worried. Some overeat because they are bored and not even hungry, others because the food is there and it shouldn't go to waste. Believe me; I know all the reasons very well. In many cases there is no need to change the diet to lose weight and keep it off: all it takes is smaller food portions and some exercise. For other people, especially when the extra fat was slow to put on, usually over years, it may be slow to come off unless major changes in diet and exercise occur. Many obesity researchers have found that significantly reducing calorie intake is most effective for weight loss. As I point out in Chapter 14, exercise is helpful but it is very difficult to exercise away body fat. It is much more efficient to avoid eating an extra 600 calories than it is to burn off 600 calories. There are some obese patients who are so overweight that exercise may be extremely difficult or even dangerous, and exercise should commence only with approval of a doctor. Once significant body fat is lost, however, exercise is essential to keep it off. Bottom line: the optimal combination is calorie reduction and exercise.

As I mentioned, controlling calorie intake is key to weight loss. High-fat diets do not necessarily cause obesity. High-calorie diets do. High-calorie diets may be high-fat diets, but they can also be low-fat, high-carbohydrate diets. Unfortunately, what too many people eat is a high-fat, high-carbohydrate, high-calorie diet, which is the worst combination for reasons I will describe in detail later (Chapter 13). A low-fat, high-carbohydrate diet of excess calories may not be good either. Accumulating evidence shows that a high-carbohydrate diet of excess calories, especially one composed of simple sugars, aggravates insulin resistance and also often increases triglyceride concentrations in the blood. What is most important is total calorie intake, not simply the fat or carbohydrate content. Fat does have twice the calorie density of carbohydrate (fat = 9.3 kilocalories per gram, or kcal/g, alcohol = 7.0 kcal/g, carbohydrate = 4.1 kcal/g; note that what food labels and diet books call a "Calorie" is equal to 1 kilocalorie of energy). There are diet strategies that substitute healthy fats for simple carbohydrates, resulting in an overall appetite reduction for many people and a total reduction in caloric intake. Although this is a controversial point, in my view dietary fat is not necessarily bad, and low-fat foods are not necessarily good, but no one can argue with the benefits of overall lower calorie intake for treating obesity.

Adipose Tissue Sends Out Signals

Most people think of body fat, as simply a mass of inert material, but in fact it is a biologically active tissue (white adipose tissue). In the mid-1990s, Jeffrey Friedman and colleagues discovered the hormone leptin (Zhang et al. 1994), whose deficiency was the apparent cause of the extreme obesity seen in a line of mutant mice known as *obese*. These mice are huge. Whereas a normal adult mouse will weigh at most 30–35 grams, my research team has seen genetically obese mice that reached 80–90 grams in weight. These mice have elevated blood lipids and severely fatty livers. They represent an extreme obesity syndrome that would translate into a person weighing around 450–500 pounds. Leptin is made by the adipose tissue. In the normal animal, leptin is secreted in proportion to adipose tissue amount; thus, when the body has stored enough energy in adipose tissue, the body fat stores send a signal to the brain via leptin that enough is enough—stop eating. This mechanism is a crucial factor in longer-term appetite control. In contrast, the feeling of a full stomach along with rising blood glucose concentrations after eating contribute to a feeling of satiety, the short-term signal to stop eating. Leptin modulates the sensitivity of the animal to signals generated during eating. *Obese* mice have a defective allele of the leptin gene such that no functional leptin is produced, resulting in a reduced feedback signal to stop eating. This becomes a powerful signal to continue eating. *Obese* mice sit in their cages in one place all of the time, usually under the food hopper, eating.

In normal animals leptin activates a region in the brain that switches off appetite and reduces food intake. Leptin also affects metabolism, especially fat metabolism. Research suggests that its effect on fat metabolism may be similar to that of the insulin-sensitizing drug, metformin (Chapter 15), in promoting fatty acid oxidation and reducing fatty acid synthesis. So in 1994, with the discovery of leptin, there was great hope that simply taking leptin would cure human obesity. Obese patients would reduce food intake and feel more energetic and their excess fat would disappear. In fact, the pharmaceutical company Amgen was counting on this and bought the drug rights to leptin. Unfortunately, most obese people already have abnormally high leptin levels, not a deficiency. Obese human patients who have a genetic deficiency of leptin are very rare, but they do respond well to leptin for weight reduction. Leptin deficiency does not appear to cause garden-variety obesity. The leptin story, however, changed our whole way of thinking about the pathophysiology of obesity.

Since leptin was discovered, many hormones and cytokines have been found that originate in white adipose tissue and that function in normal fat physiology. These include resistin, adiponectin, and tumor necrosis factor-α. So adipose tissue is not simply the "fat sink" of the body. It certainly functions in that way, but it also produces critical hormones that affect body weight through direct influences on behavior and metabolism.

Kinds of Body Fat

Adipose tissue comes in different varieties that have different properties. The first designation is between white and brown adipose tissue. White adipose tissue is the familiar fat found on a T-bone steak. In people, it is responsible for protruding bellies and enlarged buttocks. Brown adipose tissue isn't nearly as fatty as white fat because its main function is to burn fatty acids for nonshivering heat generation, and therefore it has a high density of mitochondria for energy generation. Human babies have this type adipose tissue and it may help to keep them warm. It goes away, however, as they age, and it is mostly gone by the time they become adults. Rodents have a lifelong supply of brown adipose tissue critical for thermoregulation. The importance of brown fat function was vividly demonstrated by our research team when we put mutant mice with genetically deficient fatty acid burning capabilities in a 40° F room; they could not maintain their body temperature and died. Burning fatty acids in brown fat supplies the fuel essential for nonshivering thermogenesis. Obviously, in the wild, mice rely on stores of brown fat to withstand much colder temperatures.

There are two major types of white fat, visceral adipose tissue and peripheral adipose tissue (Figure 1.1). Peripheral adipose tissue is also called subcutaneous fat. I attended the 2003 meeting of the American Diabetes Association, where I learned that there is no solid agreement about the risks of excess visceral fat versus subcutaneous fat, although most would agree that excess body fat poses significant health risks. What I describe here is a general con-

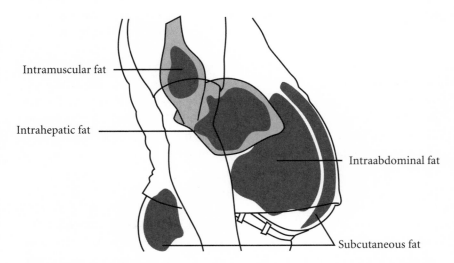

Intramuscular fat

Intrahepatic fat

Intraabdominal fat

Subcutaneous fat

Figure 1.1. Distribution of subcutaneous (peripheral) and visceral (intraabdominal) adipose tissue deposits. Internal body organs such as liver and skeletal muscle may also harbor an abnormal accumulation of intracellular fat.

sensus among many scientists about this issue. As we learn more about adipose tissue biology, the story may change.

Visceral adipose tissue, or the deeper body fat, is associated with the spaces around internal organs like the liver, intestines, and kidneys. It seems to be the type of white fat more harmful to health. It is more sensitive to catecholamines (epinephrine, norepinehrine), thus more easily stimulated for lipolysis. Lipolysis is the breaking down of the storage form of fat, known as triglyceride or triacylglycerol, into three free fatty acids and a glycerol, which then enter the blood stream. At the same time, visceral adipose tissue is also less responsive to insulin, making it easier to turn on lipolysis and harder to shut it off. If there is excess visceral fat and it tends to release fatty acids into the blood a lot of the time, insulin resistance is more likely to develop. Thus, release of fatty acids during lipolysis is beneficial if it goes for energy expenditure, but it is a problem if it is "feeding" insulin resistance.

Peripheral white adipose tissue or subcutaneous fat seems to be used more for long-term storage of fatty acids incorporated into triglycerides. It is less sensitive to the signals that promote lipolysis and more sensitive to signals, such as insulin, that oppose lipolysis. This type of fat tends to be found in the buttocks and extremities as well as around the belly. In contrast to visceral fat, found frequently in men, subcutaneous or peripheral body fat is more commonly a problem for premenopausal women. As I mentioned, this fat is less dynamic and tends to stay put. It may be what worries us most when trying on bathing suits, but metabolically it is "safer" fat than the "beer-belly" visceral type of fat. After menopause, women may become as prone to visceral adiposity as men. Obviously, these sex-influenced patterns of fat distribution are not ironclad; some women certainly have excess belly fat before menopause, and not all men get beer bellies.

One way to remember the differences between visceral adipose tissue and peripheral adipose tissue is to think about them as personal finances for the body. Visceral fat is like a checking account, easy in and easy out. Subcutaneous fat is like a retirement account, on the other hand: you may be socking it away, but it is very difficult to get back out. It has been shown that individuals who lose 5–10% of body weight may lose 30% of their visceral fat. There are significant differences in racial groups in this regard. Studies have shown that among women with the same activity level, black women have on average more peripheral fat but significantly less visceral fat than white women (Lara-Castro et al. 2002).

These different adipose tissue components are involved in the development of different disease processes. The genetic factors that affect adipose tissue function and mass are also an important part of the story.

Obesity Can Be Genetic

Some genetic changes may have a strong influence on eating and exercising behavior, so much that it seems impossible to prevent, let alone reduce, obesity in these patients. Single-gene obesity disorders such as leptin deficiency are relatively rare but easily identified, whereas more common genetic influences on obesity may be difficult to characterize. Sometimes obesity that appears to run in the family may be a consequence of everyone in that particular family having "learned" to eat a lot and exercise little—"that's what we have always done." To prove that a particular condition is genetic rather than learned, researchers study identical twins separated at birth and raised in different environments. This is an uncommon situation, but if identical twins grew up in two different environments and both ended up obese, then perhaps their obesity is genetic. If one becomes obese and the other doesn't, the "discordance" suggests that obesity in this case is not strongly influenced by genetics. From twin studies it has been estimated that heritability of BMI is 50–90% (Barsh, Farooqi, and O'Rahilly 2000). Another way to study the genetic possibility is to try to identify a specific genetic marker that appears only in the obese family members and not the lean ones. I discuss this technique in Chapter 10.

Genetic Deficiencies That Cause Inherited Obesity

Mouse mutants have given us the most genetic clues about what to look for in human obesity. Many of the "obesity" genes regulate feeding behavior. Strong biological forces must be overcome if the neurochemical pathways involved in this behavior have been disrupted. An obese mouse mutant that is similar to the leptin-deficiency mutant is deficient in leptin receptors and named the *diabetes* mutant. As you might expect, leptin deficiency would be treatable by giving leptin, but leptin receptor deficient mice have excess leptin. The problem is that the leptin molecules are unable to signal the brain cells to stop eating because the brain cells lack receptors for the molecules. Another mouse mutant, known as *obese yellow* (Figure 1.2), has a mutation that affects the pro-opiomelanocortin (POMC) pathway (Figure 1.3), which is important in reducing appetite. This mutation causes an agouti molecule to be produced in the brain that is normally made only in the skin. The aberrant production of agouti disrupts the normal function of ligands that act at the melanocortin-4 receptor, which is first signaled by leptin, and thereby produces excessive hunger. Obesity caused by the *obese yellow* mutation is an autosomal dominant trait.

Most of these mutations in mice were originally studied because they caused morbid obesity. They are all single-gene disorders that follow a Mendelian inheritance pattern. In other words, most of the disorders are recessive and will occur only if two copies of the mutant allele are inherited, one from each parent, whereas some are dominant traits that require only one mutant allele. Like many monogenic disorders, this type of obesity is powerfully influenced by single genes and resistant to environmental changes. The inherited tendency toward obesity most commonly found in people, however, is more complex, indicating that more than one gene is involved and that the environment also has a major effect on the development of body fat.

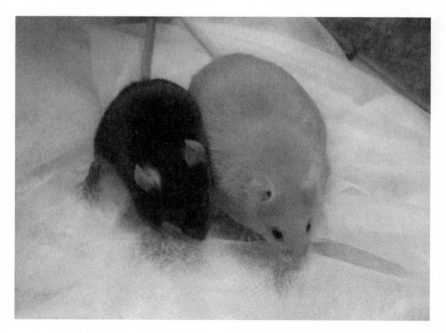

Figure 1.2. Mice with the *obese yellow* mutation have a severe form of inherited obesity. The *obese yellow* mutant on the right is twice the size of a normal mouse. (Photograph courtesy of Robert A. Kesterson.)

Genetic Deficiencies Revealed Key Mechanisms of Eating Behavior

In the brain, the region that regulates appetite and satiety is known as the hypothalamus. This is the same part of the brain that monitors and regulates, by influencing the pituitary, functions such as hormone secretion (Woods et al. 1998). It is also where leptin acts to reduce appetite by inhibiting release of another protein, neuropeptide Y (NPY) (Figure 1.3). NPY stimulates appe-

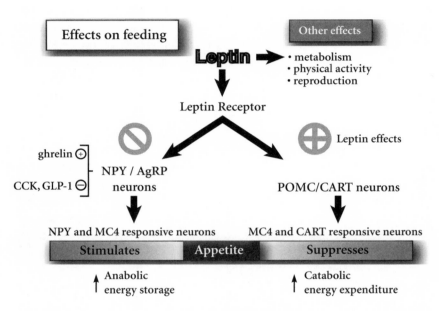

Figure 1.3. Leptin plays a central role in appetite control by either activating or inhibiting two distinct populations of neurons in the appetite center in the brain. First, leptin must interact with receptor molecules in the cell membranes of neurons. Activation by the leptin molecule will either promote or inhibit a series of reactions within the cell. In some neurons, the production of neuropeptide Y (NPY) and agouti-related peptide (AgRP), which stimulate appetite, is turned off by leptin. Acting as counterbalance is the activity of adjacent neurons that produce pro-opiomelanocortin (POMC) and cocaine and amphetamine regulated transcript (CART). These substances, which are stimulated by leptin, activate downstream neurons that actively suppress appetite. Both sides of this control mechanism—the inhibition of neurons that stimulate appetite and the activation of neurons that suppress it—are mediated by melanocortin-4 (MC4) responsive neurons through their interaction with agonists (POMC) and antagonists (AgRP). Additionally, other peptide hormones—such as the gastrointestinal peptides ghrelin, cholecystokinin (CCK), and glucagon-like peptide-1 (GLP-1)—also regulate activity of POMC/CART and NPY/AgRP neurons through their cognate receptors.

tite, and an excess of it leads to constant hunger. Normally, leptin activates the leptin receptor, which in turn inhibits the NPY neurons and at the same time activates the POMC pathway mentioned above, which reduces appetite. When this series of steps is blocked by a mutant gene, the result is constant hunger.

Appetite signaling should be in balance so that the appetite center of the brain appropriately triggers a desire to eat again when there is a negative energy balance. In a balanced system the production of NPY is stimulated when leptin concentrations drop because there has been a reduction in fat mass. In contrast, deficient activity of the NPY pathway produces anorexia. Once the appropriate amount of food has been eaten and the fat mass is restored, then the blood concentrations of leptin rise again to shut off the appetite stimulation center and eating should be reduced. Leptin, along with insulin, should be considered a long-term influence on appetite and body fat mass.

In the shorter term, such as between meals, other molecules carry signals from the digestive system that regulate feeding behavior. From the stomach comes a hormone, ghrelin, that stimulates hunger, while other digestive system hormones—such as cholecystokinin (CCK) and glucagon-like peptide (GLP-1)—reduce hunger (Flier 2004). Ghrelin is often present in high concentrations in dieters, stimulating their hunger as they try to cut back on calories. CCK and GLP-1 increase after eating to reduce hunger and subsequently food intake in the short term, independent of the increase in leptin levels due to an increase in body fat.

This is only a brief overview of a more complicated story. Furthermore, scientists are still working to understand the process of obesity. The message to take away is that obesity is intimately tied to eating behavior, which is regulated by several pathways in the brain that have been identified by the study of genetic disorders of obesity. The steps in these pathways are of great interest as drug targets.

Extremely Lean Individuals May Be Insulin Resistant

Too little adipose tissue may also be a big problem. Body fat is "good" in the right amounts in the right places. Someone with too little body fat may, like the morbidly obese individual, be severely insulin resistant. Diseases characterized by deficient adipose tissue are known as *lipodystrophy* diseases. In particular, loss of fat is called *lipoatrophy*. These diseases may be genetic, as in *lamin A* gene mutations, in which certain components of adipose tissue cells are not made, or they may be induced with certain drug therapies, such as highly active antiretroviral therapy used to treat AIDS patients.

Body fat serves the very important function of being a fatty acid "sink." That is, individuals must be able to store fatty acids as triglycerides because they will need to draw on these reserve fatty acids for energy. A bigger problem of not having adipose tissue to take up fatty acids from the blood is the buildup of fatty acids in the liver and the muscles, leading to insulin resistance.

Overall, we need the right amount of fat to act as a fatty acid sink and provide an adequate supply of fat-derived hormones and cytokines. When body fat is in excess, especially as visceral adipose tissue, it "leaks" fatty acids into the blood. Those fatty acids may accumulate in the liver and muscle, thus promoting for insulin resistance. Many of the genetic forms of obesity involve the genes that ultimately control eating behavior. Paradoxically, too little fat can cause many of the same health problems, related to insulin resistance, as does too much fat. Fundamentally, obesity is caused by excessive calorie intake relative to too little energy expenditure; in the background, genetics plays a role in both. Obesity is often associated with other diseases that share the underlying problems of excess fat in the body. Among these are excess fat stored in organs that normally do not store fat, excess lipids in the blood (including elevated triglyceride and cholesterol concentrations), as well as excess fat stored in adipose tissue. In the next chapter I cover diseases associated with excess fat.

CHAPTER 2

Testing for Silent Diseases

This chapter serves as an introductory overview of the different diseases and disease processes involving excess body fat. These include high blood lipids, insulin resistance, metabolic syndrome, and type 2 diabetes. Patients usually do not realize how serious these "silent" diseases are. Often their first indication of disease processes is the result of blood tests and other criteria commonly measured during a medical examination.

Measuring "Fatness"

A major cause of concern at a medical checkup is, of course, the amount of body fat. Patients with a protruding belly, indicating excessive stores of abdominal fat, also known as visceral obesity, are of high concern. The diseases of excess fat develop often over decades. In the United States, these disease processes are speeding up, as demonstrated by the increasing number of obese children here (and, increasingly, world-wide). Excess fat in the gut is one outward sign that disease processes involving excess body fat may already be under way. The common analogy is that those with excess fat in the butt have the figure of a pear, documented by a decreased ratio of waist-to-hip circumference (Matsuzawa 1997). In contrast, those with excess fat in the gut are said to have the shape of an apple and an increased ratio of waist-to-hip circumference. In general, it is widely considered that the pear shape is medically safer than the apple shape.

Body mass index (BMI) is used to estimate "fatness." BMI is calculated as an individual's weight (in kilograms) divided by height squared (in meters) (see Table 2.1). A normal BMI ranges from 18.5 to 25. A person with BMI of 25–30 is considered overweight. Obesity is most often defined as having a BMI greater than 30. Having a BMI of less than 18.5 is considered underweight, and this can be unhealthy as well. Overall, BMI seems to be a practical measure of "fatness" in most people; however, it gives a false representation of fatness for muscular individuals. The typical examples are the muscle-bound movie star types who have a higher BMI because they have a high muscular weight compared with their height. Individuals with an increasing BMI may already have several possible diseases processes in progress. Beyond the con-

Table 2.1. Body mass index (BMI) equals (weight in kilograms) divided by (height in meters)^2

Height in feet and inches	Weight in pounds								
	100	120	140	160	180	200	220	240	260
4′ 6″	23	28	33	37	42	47	51	56	61
4′ 7″	22	27	31	36	40	45	51	52	58
4′ 8″	22	26	30	36	39	43	47	52	56
4′ 9″	21	25	29	33	37	41	46	50	54
4′ 10″	20	24	28	32	36	40	44	48	52
4′ 11″	19	23	27	31	35	39	42	46	50
5′ 0″	19	23	26	30	34	37	41	45	49
5′ 1″	18	22	26	29	33	36	40	44	42
5′ 2″	18	21	26	28	32	35	39	42	46
5′ 3″	17	21	24	27	31	34	37	41	44
5′ 4″	17	20	23	26	30	33	36	40	43
5′ 5″	16	19	23	26	29	32	35	38	42
5′ 6″	16	18	22	25	28	31	34	37	41
5′ 7″	15	18	21	24	27	30	33	36	39
5′ 8″	15	18	21	23	26	29	32	35	38
5′ 9″	15	17	20	23	26	28	31	34	37
5′ 10″	14	17	20	22	25	28	30	33	36
5′ 11″	14	16	19	22	24	27	30	32	35
6′ 0″	13	16	19	21	24	26	29	32	34
6′ 1″	13	16	19	21	23	26	28	31	33
6′ 2″	13	15	18	20	23	25	27	30	33
6′ 3″	12	15	17	20	22	24	27	29	32
6′ 4″	12	14	17	19	22	24	26	28	31
6′ 5″	12	14	16	19	21	23	25	28	30
6′ 6″	11	14	16	18	21	23	25	27	29

spicuous presence of excess body fat, many of these disease processes are relatively silent—that is, many individuals with this body type feel fine.

The concept of having a normal BMI and then progressing to overweight and finally to obese is somewhat artificial. Disease risk is a continuum. One is not magically obese at BMI 30.01 when he or she was merely overweight at BMI 29.99. Most experts concur that overweight individuals are approaching a state of serious disease, whereas those in the obese range have arrived.

High Blood Lipids

In patients with a risk of a fat-related disease, doctors commonly check blood lipid concentrations. Most test total cholesterol, low-density lipoprotein (LDL) cholesterol, high-density lipoprotein (HDL) cholesterol, and triglycerides. It is generally considered desirable to have a total cholesterol measurement below 200 milligrams per deciliter (mg/dl), including both LDL and HDL cholesterol. Unfortunately, as people age and increase in girth, the pattern tends toward higher concentrations of triglycerides, total, and LDL cholesterol and lower concentrations of HDL cholesterol, especially in overweight and obese people.

Having excess blood lipids is called *hyperlipidemia,* which frequently includes high blood cholesterol concentrations *(hypercholesterolemia)* and high blood triglyceride concentrations *(hypertriglyceridemia).* These two conditions may occur together or individually. An individual's current level of fatness, activity, diet, hormone status, as well as genetics and age all influence both conditions. The dangers of hyperlipidemia may also include atherosclerosis and pancreatitis, as described in Chapter 4.

High Blood Glucose

Frequently, blood glucose concentration is also measured at an annual checkup. The test is often called a "fasting blood sugar." For too many, the blood glucose concentration may be easing on up over 100 mg/dl, exceeding the 80–95 mg/dl range defined as "normal" by most laboratories. A rising blood glucose concentration is one of the first hints of possible insulin resistance.

When blood glucose is above the normal range, beta cells in the Islets of Langerhans in the pancreas are putting out extra insulin because insulin is fighting an uphill battle, known as insulin resistance, to get the body's cells to take up glucose at the normal rate. Now blood insulin concentrations begin to rise and blood glucose drops back to the normal range. This is not diabetes ... yet.

Metabolic syndrome ensues from insulin resistance. Metabolic syndrome begins as insulin resistance but also includes some or all of the following characteristics: high blood pressure *(hypertension)*, abnormal blood clotting *(dysfibrinolysis)*, excess fat storage in the liver cells *(hepatosteatosis)*, excessive fat in muscle cells, small, dense LDL particles in the blood, hypertriglyceridemia, and low HDL cholesterol. Metabolic syndrome (also known as syndrome X and insulin resistance syndrome) is a common predecessor to type 2 diabetes, a heart attack, or both (Reaven, Strom, and Fox 2000). This syndrome is described in detail in Chapter 5. I will leave until Chapter 6 a more detailed discussion of the differences between insulin-dependent (type 1) diabetes mellitus and noninsulin-dependent (type 2) diabetes.

A major frustration I hear from many people interested in learning about these disease processes is that the medical terms and abbreviations are hard to understand and that there is too much jargon in most of the medical literature. In the next chapter, I take that issue head on.

CHAPTER 3

An Introduction to the Terminology

In order to understand the various diseases of excess fat, you must first learn about the different types of fat and their properties. This chapter introduces terms and abbreviations that will help you understand the chapters to follow.

Quick Definitions

Body mass index (BMI), remember, is an estimate of fatness calculated as body weight (kg) divided by the square of body height (m²). A person with BMI of 25–30 is considered overweight, while a BMI over 30 is the definition of obesity. People sometimes speak of having "slow metabolism" and say that is why they are obese. What they are likely referring to is their *resting energy expenditure* (REE) and whether it is low or high. REE is the energy the body expends when at rest; it is also called *resting metabolic rate* (RMR). It is the body's background energy expenditure or release occurring all the time, even during sleep. People with a relatively large muscle mass tend to have a higher REE, while obese individuals of the same weight but with relatively less muscle mass have a lower REE. I will discuss energy expenditure further in Chapter 14, on exercise.

Nonalcoholic steatohepatitis (NASH) is a term heard much more frequently than in the past because it is often associated with obesity. It literally means excessive fat in the liver with inflammation and it is not caused by excessive alcohol intake. This is distinctly different from the commonly recognized alcoholic liver disease that may progress to cirrhosis. I will cover NASH in more detail in Chapter 5.

Glycemic index (GI) is a measure of how quickly digested foods containing carbohydrates are absorbed into the bloodstream and raise the concentration of blood sugar, or glucose. Simple sugars like glucose and sucrose—which splits into its constituent parts of glucose and fructose—have a high glycemic index. These sugars are readily absorbed, and the glucose in the blood stimulates insulin secretion. Foods with more complex carbohydrates, such as starch, may also have a high GI. A diet high in high-GI foods may be an underlying problem in development of insulin resistance, as explained in Chapter 13. In contrast, foods high in fiber, another dietary carbohydrate, have a low GI, and fat, which does not break down into glucose, has a GI of zero.

Anatomy of Fat

Fat is the chief form of energy storage in the body. Fat tissue is also known as *adipose tissue* and is composed of cells called *adipocytes*. These cells store predominantly triglycerides, one of many types of lipid molecules. Lipids are a group of essential compounds that are water insoluble. Being insoluble in water, lipids cannot be carried in the bloodstream unless they are modified or combined with other molecules, usually proteins.

The most famous lipids are cholesterol and triglycerides, but these large molecules may break into component parts (like fatty acids) or join with other molecules to form compounds. Most people are somewhat familiar with these terms because their blood concentrations of total cholesterol and triglycerides have been measured as part of a medical exam. Other measures include the so-called bad cholesterol, also known as low-density lipoprotein (LDL) cholesterol, and the good cholesterol, high-density lipoprotein (HDL) cholesterol. Lipoproteins are complexes of lipids and proteins that allow the water-insoluble lipids to be carried in the blood.

Cholesterol

Cholesterol is often portrayed as a "bad" lipid, but it is essential for life. Cholesterol, not officially a fat molecule but a sterol (an alcohol molecule made from a type of lipid molecule), is required in cell membranes and is essential for hormone synthesis, to mention just two of its vital functions. The problems arise when too much cholesterol ends up in the wrong place at the wrong time, clogging blood vessels or forming gallstones. Humans synthesize around

0.5 to 0.75 grams of cholesterol per day, and may take in an additional 0.25 to 0.5 grams per day in the diet. Overall it is generally understood that there is approximately a 1 gram influx of cholesterol per day. Cholesterol is a multi-ringed molecule (Figure 3.1) that is insoluble in water. A waxy substance, it is normally found in cell membranes, where it makes the membrane more rigid. Cholesterol is a compact molecule, and when positioned as part of a cell membrane it "stiffens" the membrane. This stiffness promotes compression of membrane lipids, thus reducing fluidity or flexibility. In the normal, controlled situation, this stiffness is required for normal function of the cell membrane. Free cholesterol found in cell membranes is the most abundant form of cholesterol in the body.

Another form of cholesterol is the cholesterol ester, which is a regular cholesterol molecule with an additional fatty acid molecule on one end (Figure 3.1). The attachment of the fatty acid makes it more hydrophobic, thus allowing it to have a co-existence with triglycerides. These modified cholesterol molecules are structurally normal and are required in healthy amounts as a means for transport in the blood. Once cholesterol esters stray from the bloodstream, they become the villains of our story.

Cholesterol becomes a problem when its blood concentration is greater than 200 mg/dl. This measurement refers to the total cholesterol that is contained within the lipid transport complexes found in the blood, the lipoproteins. Thus, knowing the total blood cholesterol concentration is helpful,

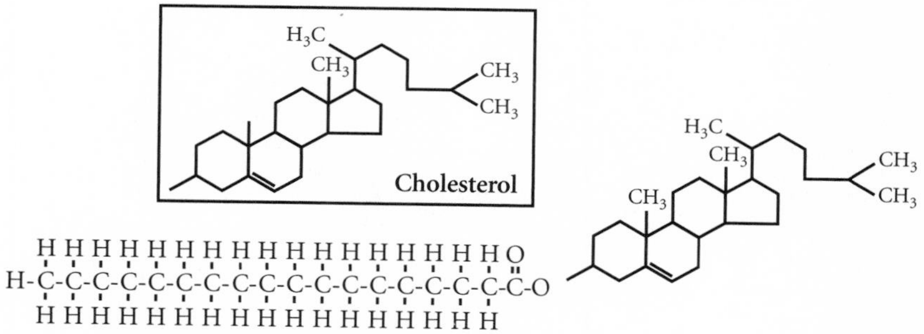

Cholesterol ester = cholesterol + fatty acid (Stearate)

Figure 3.1. Cholesterol and cholesterol ester. Free cholesterol (*above*) is converted into cholesterol ester by attachment of a fatty acid. Free cholesterol in cell membranes is the most common form in the entire body, while cholesterol ester is the most common form of cholesterol in the blood lipoproteins.

but it is only an estimate of the whole body's cholesterol status and does not tell the whole story. Often in addition to total cholesterol, what we want to know is the proportion of cholesterol in the "bad" LDL fraction and that contained in the "good" HDL fraction. There are other cholesterol-containing lipoprotein fractions as well, such as *chylomicrons*, VLDL *(very low density lipoprotein)*, and IDL *(intermediate-density lipoprotein)*. These others are not routinely measured but can be very important in evaluating and treating a condition known as dyslipidemia or hyperlipidemia, which involves abnormally high amounts of the different lipids in the blood.

Fatty Acids

Fatty acids not only build up in the blood and body tissues in people with diseases like diabetes mellitus, but these compounds can also be markedly influenced by dietary intake of fats and carbohydrates from different sources. That

Fatty acid - "saturated" 18 carbon length

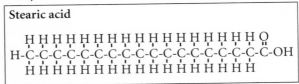

Fatty acid - "unsaturated" 18 carbon length

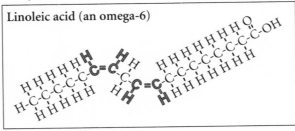

Figure 3.2. The flexibility of fatty acids is primarily determined by the type of bonds between carbons. "Saturated" fatty acids *(above)* have no double bonds between adjacent carbons, which are organized in a straight chain. "Unsaturated" fatty acids *(below)* have double bonds that put "kinks" in the structure; they are more loosely packed than the compact saturated molecules and have a lower melting temperature. The hydrogens in gray are in the *cis* position (side by side). Linoleic acid is classified as an omega-6 fatty acid because the first double bond occurs at the sixth carbon from the end.

is, the types of fatty acids that are in the blood and stored in body fat are affected by the types of fats that are eaten. A lot of information has been in the news recently concerning the undesirable health effects of saturated and *trans* fats. In contrast, there may be health advantages to consuming unsaturated fats. Some fatty acids are essential for health because mammalian cells are incapable of synthesizing them and they must be obtained from the diet. I will return to this subject after first presenting the structures of fatty acids.

Fatty acids (Figure 3.2) are the building blocks of stored fat, the lipid triglyceride or triacylglycerol. Triglycerides are composed of three fatty acids attached to a glycerol backbone. A fatty acid is a molecule composed of carbon-hydrogen units with an acid structure (–COOH) on one end (Figure 3.2). A fatty acid is unsaturated if there is a double bond between the carbon-hydrogen units (Figure 3.2). Saturated fatty acids have no double bonds, making them straight, tightly packed molecules (Figure 3.2), somewhat like cholesterol. Unsaturated fatty acids contain one or more double bonds in the *cis* (side-by-side) configuration. *Monounsaturated fatty acids* (MUFAs) have one double bond; *polyunsaturated fatty acids* (PUFAs) have two or more double bonds (Table 3.1).

Monounsaturated fatty acids are desirable and common in the diet. In Figure 3.2 (lower panel) the polyunsaturated fatty acid linoleic acid is shown. Another common and important monounsaturated fatty acid, found in olive oil and macadamia nut oil, is oleic acid. Some of the PUFAs are also important as essential fatty acids, as well as the health-promoting fatty acids found in fish known as omega-3 fatty acids (see below). The type of chemical bond

Table 3.1. Common dietary fatty acids

Fatty acid name (common dietary source)	Carbon chain length: number of double bonds	Naming by omega terminology
Palmitic acid (animal and plant fats)	$C_{16:0}$	—
Stearic acid (animal fats)	$C_{18:0}$	—
Oleic acid (animal fats, olive oil)	$C_{18:1}$	omega-9
Linoleic acid (plant oils)	$C_{18:2}$	omega-6
α-Linolenic acid (plant oils)	$C_{18:3}$	omega-3
Arachidonic acid (plant oils)	$C_{20:4}$	omega-6
Eicosapentaenoic acid (EPA) (fish oil)	$C_{20:5}$	omega-3
Docosahexaenoic acid (DHA) (fish oil)	$C_{22:6}$	omega-3

Note: Omega terminology indicates which carbon from the methyl-end of the chain has the first double bond; saturated fatty acids, with no double bonds, therefore have no name in omega terminology.

in a molecule may not sound very important, but this property determines whether a particular fat is liquid or solid at room temperature, as well as what its properties will be within the human body.

Many people erroneously think that vegetable-derived fat, like corn oil, is 100% unsaturated fat and that an animal-derived fat is 100% saturated fat. Actually, no dietary fat is all saturated or all unsaturated; all dietary fats are a mixture of two types of fatty acids (Figure 3.3), and it is the predominant percentages that are used to characterize a fat one way or another. For example, corn oil has a very high percentage of unsaturated fatty acids (>85%), which means it has lots of fatty acids with double bonds and is liquid at room temperature. Lard, though, is solid because it contains a relatively higher proportion of saturated fatty acids (>32%) and cholesterol. The character of the fats one eats affects the character of the fat deposited in one's blood vessels and adipose tissues. Saturated fatty acids that make up saturated fat, like those fats found in meats or dairy products, are straight-chain molecules with relatively high melting temperatures and are considered undesirable. Unsaturated fats have lower melting points, are liquid at room temperature, and remain so even at refrigerator temperatures. These fats have lower melting temperatures because the presence of double bonds introduces bends or kinks (Figure 3.2)

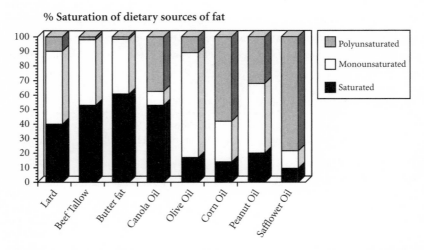

Figure 3.3. Dietary fats contain a mixture of saturated and unsaturated fatty acids (Data from Durkee, Inc., "Typical Compositions and Chemical Constants of Common Edible Fats and Oils," received August 13, 1997.)

in the fatty acid molecules, making them pack together with less density. Thus, plant-derived oils (corn oil, soybean oil, canola oil, olive oil, etc.) tend to have a much higher percentage of unsaturated fatty acids, while animal-derived oils (beef tallow, milk fat, lard) tend to be more saturated. Again, neither is purely one or the other. For example, corn oil is approximately 85% unsaturated (mono-, di-, and polyunsaturates), but it also contains approximately 15% saturated fatty acids, mostly palmitic (C_{16}) acid. Lard contains approximately 35% saturated fatty acids, mostly palmitic acid, but it also contains 65% unsaturated fatty acids.

Another type of fat that has been in the news is *trans* fatty acids, which are used to "stiffen" food products such as margarine, shortening, and peanut butter. *Trans* fats are commonly used to make margarines spreadable, like butter, and they also reduce rancidification. In chemistry, *trans* means "across from." *Trans* fatty acids are produced by *hydrogenating* unsaturated fats: by adding hydrogen, the fatty acid's double bonds are reduced to single bonds, such that the fatty acid becomes more saturated, or the hydrogens are rearranged so that there is still a double bond, making it still unsaturated, but the hydrogens are diagonally across from each other—in a *trans* rather than a *cis* arrangement. The *cis* orientation produces the kink in the molecule (Figure 3.2—lower). *Trans* hydrogens make the fatty acid a straight molecule with no kink (Figure 3.4—upper). Despite being derived from vegetable sources and being an unsaturated fatty acid, *trans* fatty acids have virtually all of the characteristics of a saturated fatty acid (Figure 3.4—upper), including a high melting temperature. In addition, evidence is increasing that consumption of *trans* fatty acids has most, if not more, of the detrimental properties of eating animal-derived saturated fats.

Another category of fatty acids that we hear about is the *omega fatty acids* (Figure 3.4—lower), usually in discussions about increasing our consumption of fish or adding fish oil supplements to the diet. The term *omega* refers to which carbon from the end of the unsaturated fatty acid molecule has the first double bond. One of two omega fatty acids frequently associated with fish is eicosapentaenoic acid (EPA), an omega-3 fatty acid that is 20 carbons in length with 5 double bonds, the most outside bond being 3 carbons from the end position. The second fish-derived omega-3 fatty acid is docosahexaenoic acid (DHA) (Figure 3.4), a 22-carbon fatty acid with 6 double bonds. Other omega fatty acids commonly found in the diet include oleic (omega-9), linoleic (omega-6), linolenic (omega-3), and arachidonic (omega-6) fatty acids.

Scientists are currently investigating whether omega-3 dietary fatty acids may help decrease a person's risk of certain types of cancer, whereas omega-6 fatty acids may not.

Although the body can synthesize fatty acids and many other lipids from dietary carbohydrates, animals' diets must still provide certain fatty acids that are derived from plant sources. These are known as *essential* fatty acids: linoleic, linolenic, and arachidonic fatty acids. Animal cells can synthesize only relatively simple fatty acids, predominantly of the saturated variety. For full health, humans require relatively small amounts of the more complex fatty acids with numerous double bonds that our cells are incapable of producing. What makes these fatty acids essential is not fully understood, but it is known that they are required for synthesis of prostaglandins, prostacyclins, and thromboxanes required for inflammatory responses to infection, skin health, platelet function, and other processes. For example, prostaglandins function by activating cellular processes at very low concentrations, and they have a very short half-life (30 seconds to a few minutes at most).

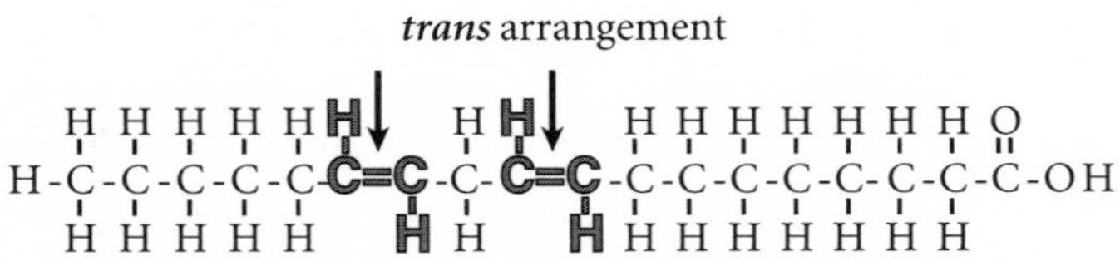

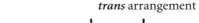

trans arrangement

Linoleic acid (an omega-6 fatty acid from plant oils)

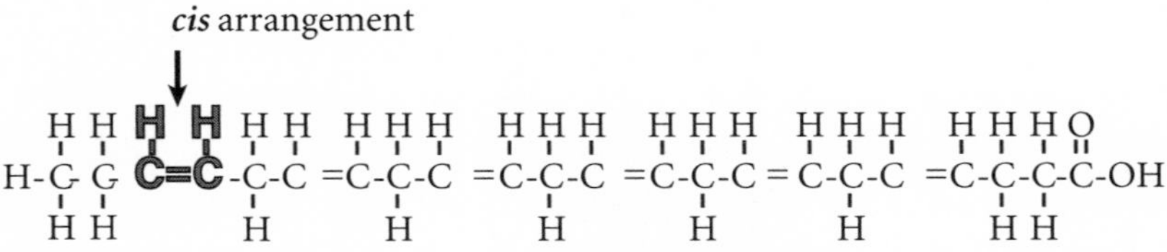

cis arrangement

Docosahexaenoic acid (DHA) (an omega-3 fatty acid from fish oil)

Figure 3.4. The distinguishing features of a *trans* versus a *cis* arrangement in fatty acids are demonstrated by the double bonds indicated by the arrows. In a *trans* fatty acid *(above),* the hydrogens attached to the carbons joined by double bonds are diagonally across from each other. In contrast, in a *cis* fatty acid *(below),* the hydrogens are arranged side by side. Note that the only difference between the linoleic acid shown here and the linoleic acid in Figure 3.2 is the arrangement of the hydrogens, which changes the shape of the molecule and therefore its chemical properties (such as melting temperature).

Triglycerides

Triglycerides (Figure 3.5), also known as triacylglycerols, are the building blocks of stored fat in adipose tissue, as well as the predominant form of fat in foods. They also compose the fat that builds up in tissues during the disease processes to be discussed in this book. These lipid molecules can be broken down *(lipolysis)* in the adipose tissues during periods of fasting or starvation to provide fatty acids as metabolic fuel, used especially by the liver and by the skeletal and heart muscle. Triglycerides are carried in the blood predominantly in chylomicrons (after eating) and VLDL (fasting) particles. People

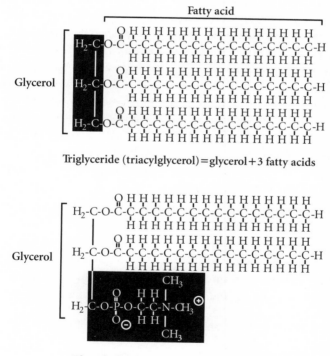

Figure 3.5. Triglyceride *(above)* has a glycerol backbone (highlighted) with three fatty acids attached. A phospholipid *(below)* has a similar structure except for a phosphate group (highlighted) in place of a fatty acid. The phospholipid shown here, phosphatidylcholine, has attached to its phosphate group the alcohol choline.

whose blood triglycerides are over 200 mg/dl have a condition known as hypertriglyceridemia. Some patients may have concentrations even higher, over 1,000 mg/dl, at which time they become at high risk for pancreatitis, an inflammatory disease of the pancreas. Excess VLDL particles are considered a significant health risk, just as excess LDL cholesterol concentrations are.

Phospholipids and Glycolipids

Fat molecules come in many different forms that serve different functions in different parts of the cell. For energy storage in the form of fat, uncharged, hydrophobic triglycerides function well. For fat molecules to be able to interact with other molecules, such as adjacent proteins or ions in the water environment, they require specialized components that provide a charge to their molecular structure. Some lipid molecules may play a role in cellular signaling or binding ions, such as calcium. The phospholipids and glycolipids are examples of lipids that have specialized functions beyond energy storage. All the cell membranes in the body contain phospholipids and glycolipids in various combinations, depending on the needed fluidity properties of the given cell.

Phospholipids are especially important in cell membranes and lipoproteins (Figure 3.5). These molecules look much like triglycerides but have a modification at one of the three positions that is usually occupied by a fatty acid: the addition of a phosphate group. This modification makes the lipid have a charge, unlike any of the other lipids described thus far. The closely related glycolipids are somewhat similar in form and function to phospholipids, but they contain a sugar component rather than a phosphate group. You may have heard of one of the glycolipid groups, the gangliosides, because it is this class of lipids that build up and cause the fatal disease of children known as Tay-Sachs disease. In the cell membrane, both phospholipids and glycolipids are arranged in a bilayer form. It is the optimal combination of cholesterol, phospholipids, glycolipids, and various proteins that make a cell membrane functional.

The lipids group of compounds consists mainly of cholesterol, free fatty acids, or fatty acids incorporated into triglycerides, cholesterol esters, phospholipids and glycolipids. They are predominantly water-insoluble compounds that have a wide range of "packing" properties. These properties, which depend on carbon chain length (long or short structures) and the number of double bonds, determine the flexibility and melting properties of the lipid mixture. Their combined properties make lipids essential to normal mammalian biology, but deadly if they accumulate in the wrong places in concentrations that are too high. One goal of many diets and drug therapies is to regulate, usually to lower, these lipids in the blood, thus reducing the deposition of fat in undesirable places, such as the arteries.

In the next chapters I will elaborate on the disease processes that may occur when blood lipid concentrations reach abnormally high levels.

CHAPTER 4

Disorders of Excess Cholesterol and Triglycerides

In this chapter I introduce the common disorders of elevated blood lipids that develop as people age. Although there are distinct genetic diseases of cholesterol metabolism such as familial hypercholesterolemia, the most common forms of hypercholesterolemia have no clear genetic patterns associated with them. Certainly, genetic components influence these common lipid disorders, but they have their effect by a subtle and complex interaction among multiple genes, which is further affected by environmental factors like diet and exercise.

Fats are essential for life, but in the wrong place or the wrong form, they can cause disease. Cholesterol, for example, occurs in many forms and in many parts of the body, for better or for worse. This chapter follows the adventures of cholesterol throughout the body and the diseases it may cause.

Where Does Cholesterol Come From?

A multiring molecule of the sterol family of compounds, cholesterol is insoluble in water but is soluble in fat. Because it is fat soluble, it is often grouped with the fats or lipids. Cholesterol with a fatty acid attached at one end is a cholesterol ester. This is the most common form of cholesterol in the blood. Since cholesterol is a waxy material and will not dissolve in the blood, which is predominantly water, it must be transported by structures known as lipoproteins. Lipoproteins are important to understand because of their effect on health: low-density lipoproteins (LDL) are considered "bad" for health and high-density lipoproteins (HDL) are the "good" cholesterol.

Cholesterol can be synthesized by the body or obtained from the diet.

Ideally, when the body's needs are met through diet, the body's synthesis decreases accordingly and the resulting blood concentration remains normal. The single most commonly used criterion in evaluating the body's cholesterol status is in the blood concentration of total cholesterol. That concentration is not the whole picture, but it portrays enough of the scene for explanatory purposes. First, let's consider the amounts we are talking about here. The net influx—that is, intake plus synthesis—is only about 0.25–1 gram of cholesterol per day. One gram is equal in weight to about a third of a teaspoon of water—not much. In contrast, a person's total fat intake per day may be as high as 40–150 grams. An entire stick of margarine (8 tablespoons) contains 80 grams of fat. An average egg has about 0.25 gram (250 mg) of cholesterol. Studies have found that human subjects absorbed only about 38–81% of the cholesterol they ingested, and the absorption is potentially further reduced by ingestion of plant sterols that have a molecular structure similar to that of cholesterol (Grundy, Ahrens, and Davignon 1969). Thus, the amount of cholesterol involved is a relatively small proportion of total lipid intake, yet it is the most well known type of lipid in the body. Most people know what their blood cholesterol concentrations are, but they likely do not know their blood triglyceride concentrations. Knowing both is important.

Internal Synthesis of Cholesterol

Although the liver is central to maintaining a regulatory role for flux of cholesterol around the body, most cholesterol is produced in other organs. Virtually all cells are capable of cholesterol synthesis and require no extracellular source. In most species, 60–85% of total body cholesterol synthesis is accounted for outside the liver (Dietschy 1997). Liver exports cholesterol in order to produce VLDL particles capable of triglyceride efflux. Crucial amounts of cholesterol are produced for steroid hormone synthesis in the adrenal glands, testes, or ovaries. Cholesterol synthesis is a highly regulated process. As scientists decode the individual steps and their regulation, effective drugs may be developed to help control blood cholesterol levels.

The collective research of Konrad Bloch, Feodor Lynen, John Cornforth, G. Popjak, and Robert Woodward, early pioneers in this field, contributed a great deal to our understanding cholesterol synthesis (Bloch 1965). Cholesterol is synthesized from acetyl coenzyme A (acetyl-CoA) in a multistep process. Acetyl-CoA is a final end product from the complete metabolism of sugar (glucose) and from oxidation of fatty acids. The majority of acetyl-CoA for cholesterol synthesis probably comes from glucose. It is necessary to understand a few chemical intermediates in this process so that later discussions of cholesterol-lowering drugs will make sense.

Figure 4.1 outlines the key points of cholesterol synthesis. Acetyl-CoA goes through two steps to become β-hydroxy-β-methylglutaryl-CoA (HMG-CoA). The next step, in which HMG-CoA is converted to mevalonate by the enzyme HMG-CoA reductase, is the rate-limiting step of cholesterol synthesis. In other words, this is the step that determines the rate of cholesterol synthesis, and if we can regulate that step, we should have a significant effect on cholesterol synthesis. There are more than a dozen additional steps in this process, but this one must be emphasized because it is inhibition at this step that is key for the action of the so-called statin drugs, or HMG-CoA reductase inhibitors. You are likely familiar with medicines such as lovastatin (Mevacor), ator-

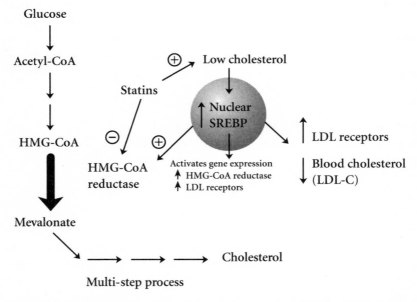

Figure 4.1. Abbreviated diagram of the steps of cholesterol synthesis and its regulation. The action of HMG-CoA reductase in converting HMG-CoA to mevalonate is key in regulating cholesterol synthesis. Statins inhibit this enzyme, so it is not available to do its part in synthesizing cholesterol. A reduction in cholesterol in turn increases the sterol-response element binding protein (SREBP) in the nucleus of cells, which increases expression of LDL receptors. With more receptors in its cell membrane, the cell will bring more LDLs from the blood into the cell, thereby reducing the LDL cholesterol concentration in the blood.

vastatin (Lipitor), rousavastatin (Crestor), simvastatin (Zocor), pravastatin (Pravachol), and fluvastatin (Lescol). I will devote an entire chapter (Chapter 15) to discussing the various drugs used for lowering cholesterol and how they work.

This rate-limiting step requires HMG-CoA reductase, a finely tuned enzyme. An intracellular "cholesterol thermostat" monitors the concentration of sterols or cholesterol-like molecules, such that when cholesterol or sterols are high, this system signals the HMG-CoA reductase gene in the cell nucleus to decrease the amount of HMG-CoA reductase being synthesized. The effect is a reduction of cholesterol synthesis. Therefore, the cell will turn down or turn off completely the synthesis when there is already plenty of cholesterol around. So to a certain extent, when external supplies of cholesterol are present, the cells should be signaled to quit the internal synthesis of cholesterol. The intracellular system that monitors cholesterol levels involves the sterol response element binding protein (SREBP), and its associated proteins together carry out this elegant regulatory process (Brown and Goldstein 1997). SREBP is the signal molecule that will be freed up to go to the cell's nucleus to activate the HMG-CoA reductase gene when more cholesterol is needed. It gets its name because it binds to a regulatory element of the HMG-CoA reductase gene and other genes that encode for enzymes involved in cholesterol synthesis. This binding activates the expression of these enzymes in order to increase cholesterol synthesis during times of low intracellular cholesterol. If sterols are already high or sufficient in the cell, SREBP remains firmly attached to the inside of the cell and does not go to the nucleus, where the gene targets are located.

Another major player in this process of cholesterol regulation is the LDL receptor, which is extremely important for the import of cholesterol into cells, such as hepatocytes. The cholesterol contained within LDL particles is what tends to accumulate in blood-derived cells known as macrophages. The mechanisms are not entirely clear; however, it appears LDL particles are modified in some way that makes them attractive for loading into macrophages. Cholesterol-filled macrophages play an important role in the clogging of arteries. While SREBP is regulating the production of cholesterol-synthesizing enzymes, it also regulates the expression of LDL receptor molecules; the quantity of LDL receptors available on the cell surface will determine how many LDL particles will be pulled from the blood into the cell. When intracellular cholesterol is high, there is a reduction in the number of LDL receptors so that less and less cholesterol will be brought into the cell from the blood LDLs. Thus, the cell's net response to reduced SREBP activity is to reduce synthesis of cholesterol (by reducing the amount of enzymes available to carry out the synthesis steps) and, at the same time, to reduce the amount of cholesterol that is being imported via the LDL receptor on the cell surface. The overall effect is that the hepatocyte's uptake of LDL cholesterol from the blood is reduced, resulting in a greater amount of LDL cholesterol in the blood.

Lipoproteins: Cholesterol and Triglycerides

The digestion of dietary fat starts in the stomach and upper small intestine. While in the upper small intestine, the digesting food is mixed with bile, coming from the gallbladder, and digestive enzymes, such as the *lipases* (enzymes that break down lipids), coming from the pancreas. The bile and pancreatic enzymes are secreted into the small intestine through ducts. As the digesting food breaks down, the cholesterol and fatty acids originally making up the food fats are freed and absorbed into the intestinal mucosa. These absorbed lipid components are formed by the mucosal cells into large particles containing both proteins and lipids, the *chylomicrons* that pass into the lymphatics and eventually the bloodstream via the thoracic duct. The whole set of lipid-carrying particles found in the blood are known as *lipoproteins.*

The lipid in chylomicrons, primarily triglyceride with some cholesterol, is next taken up mostly by tissues other than the liver. An enzyme, *lipoprotein lipase,* found in the capillaries of heart, adipose tissue, spleen, kidney, and other tissues, but not liver, helps extract the fatty acids (>90%) that make up the triglycerides contained within the chylomicron. Depending on the organ, the cells receiving the fatty acids will either metabolize them for energy production (e.g., skeletal and heart muscle) or store them by forming new triglycerides (as occurs in adipose tissues). The remaining cholesterol components from the chylomicron remnants eventually pass into the liver cells via the chylomicron remnant uptake mechanism.

When fatty acids build up as triglycerides in the liver, hepatocytes export them by forming *very low density lipoproteins* (VLDLs). VLDLs, like chylomicrons, also provide fatty acids to cells. In general, chylomicrons provide fatty acids to the adipose tissues and VLDLs provide fatty acids to skeletal muscle and the heart. Thus, dietary fatty acids have a direct route to adipose tissue, the storage site. Having high blood triglycerides usually means that VLDL concentration is abnormally high, if the blood was sampled after fasting. High blood triglycerides can also be the result of excessive chylomicron concentrations, which commonly occur after consumption of a high-fat meal.

All of the lipoproteins contain cholesterol, but chylomicrons and VLDLs are the largest and most buoyant in water because each lipoprotein contains a high proportion of lipid. Chylomicrons and VLDLs are composed of triglyceride and cholesterol but also the "starter" proteins known as apolipoproteins, in particular *apolipoprotein B* (apoB for short), *apolipoprotein E* (apoE), and *apolipoprotein C-II* (apoC-II). Chylomicrons differ slightly from VLDLs because they are assembled in the intestine; the apoB in the chylomicron structure is a shorter form (known as apoB-48 because it is only 48% of the size of the apoB-100 produced by the liver for VLDL synthesis). Since lipids are insoluble in water or blood, they must be combined with carrier proteins to move around the body in the bloodstream. The apolipoproteins facilitate movement of lipids in the blood and act as targeting molecules so that the lipids being transported in the blood end up in the right places.

The apolipoproteins are categorized into two major groups on the basis of their functional properties. Some apolipoproteins are structural, meaning that they are an essential component of the fully constituted lipoprotein, while others are exchangeable among lipoproteins. ApoB-48 of chylomicrons and apoB-100 of VLDL, *intermediate-density lipoprotein* (IDL, which is "intermediate" in density between VLDLs and LDLs), and LDL, as well as apoA-I in HDL, are all essential components of these lipoproteins. In contrast, apolipoproteins such as apoC, apoD, and apoE are exchangeable among lipoproteins. Lipoproteins can be separated by agarose gel electrophoresis techniques into classes by density: chylomicrons (density < 0.96), β-lipoproteins (LDL density $1.006–1.063$), pre–β-lipoproteins (VLDL density < 1.006), and α-lipoproteins (HDL density $1.063–1.21$), as measured by comparison with the density of water, 1.000 g/ml (Mayes 2000). Figure 4.2 and Table 4.1 show the different lipoprotein classes, their main lipid cargo, and where each is going.

As VLDLs make their way in the blood, they are reduced to the next form, intermediate-density lipoprotein (IDL), as lipoprotein lipase, the enzyme found in capillary beds outside the liver, gradually "whittles away" at the triglyceride found in the VLDL. This process of breaking down triglycerides frees up fatty acids that can be used for energy by these tissues and, at the same time, reduces the proportion of triglyceride in the lipoprotein. Although the triglyceride content is lower than that of VLDLs, an excess of IDL is considered unhealthy because of its potential for causing atherosclerosis. As the triglyc-

eride content of these lipoproteins drops and the relative amount of cholesterol increases, these particles become a low-density lipoprotein. By now they
have lost a majority of triglyceride and apoE and their main cargo is cholesterol. LDL cholesterol is readily available to accumulate in the cardiovascular
system. LDL is even more atherogenic when it is attached to another molecule—*apolipoprotein-a,* or apo(a), often called apo "little" a. This combination
is known as *Lp(a).* So individuals with high Lp(a) have the most potentially
"bad" LDL cholesterol.

LDL-derived cholesterol is the major source of cholesterol deposits in the
arteries, known as *plaques.* Plaques appear to form as the tissue scavenger
cells—the macrophages—become overloaded with cholesterol and begin accumulating in arteries. It is widely accepted that this accumulation initiates

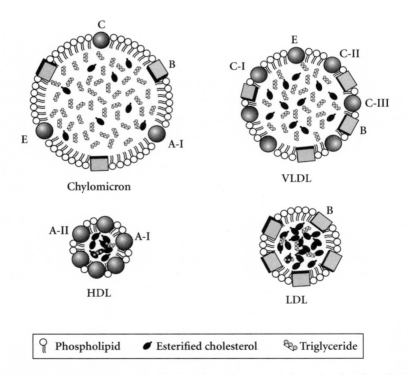

Figure 4.2. Lipoproteins are molecular complexes that carry cholesterol and triglyceride in
the blood. The relative size and constituent components are demonstrated. The large molecules in the outer phospholipid layer are apolipoproteins, which serve as targets for cellular
receptors. See also Table 4.1. (Figure courtesy of Jere P. Segrest.)

Table 4.1. Lipoproteins, from the largest and most buoyant to the smallest and most dense

Lipoprotein	Major lipid (apolipoprotein types)	Tissue of origin	Target tissue
Chylomicrons	Dietary triglyceride; cholesterol ester (A-I, A-II, C-I, C-II, C-III, E, B)	Intestine	Nonliver tissues
VLDL	Endogenous triglyceride (C-I, C-II, C-III, E, B)	Liver	Nonliver tissues
IDL	Triglyceride (B, E)	Liver (from VLDL)	Nonliver tissues
LDL	Cholesterol ester (B)	Liver (from IDL)	Nonliver tissues
HDL	Cholesterol ester (A-I, A-II, E, C-I, C-II, C-III)	Assembled in blood	Liver

inflammatory processes that end up as what we know as atherosclerosis. Excess LDL and VLDL often make up a majority of the cholesterol lipoprotein fractions in the blood of persons with pathologically high blood cholesterol levels.

Finally, there is the "good" cholesterol fraction, the high-density lipoprotein (HDL). HDL is considered the lipoprotein essential for movement of cholesterol away from or out of tissues and back to the liver for eventual disposal. People with low HDL cholesterol fractions tend to be at higher risk for cardiovascular disease; when combined with abnormally high LDL cholesterol, the risk is even greater. Premenopausal women often have a more favorable lipoprotein distribution (high HDL cholesterol and low LDL cholesterol) and overall lower total cholesterol concentrations than do men or postmenopausal women. Knowing these fractions is important because the relative amounts have consequences for health. A person with a total cholesterol concentration of 160 mg/dl might be considered healthy, but not if 120 mg/dl is contained in the LDL fraction and only 25 mg/dl is contained in the HDL fraction (with the remainder being found in other lipoproteins such as VLDL). Such a person is at risk for cardiovascular disease because the predominant form of cholesterol is the type that is deposited in the tissues and very little is on its way to elimination.

Another important concept to learn as we go over these diseases in general is that total blood cholesterol is simply a measurement of the total cholesterol in the blood without regard to specific lipoprotein fraction (LDL, HDL, etc.). More specialized tests are required to determine the actual amounts of cholesterol in the LDL fraction or the HDL fraction. So when I mention that LDL is abnormally high, I will mean that LDL cholesterol is abnormally high. Cholesterol is not free in the blood. Remember, cholesterol is insoluble in water, and blood is mostly water. Also realize that triglycerides in the blood are mostly contained within chylomicrons, which are produced from digesting foods, and VLDLs, which are produced from molecules that have been transported to the liver. When I mention high blood triglyceride concentrations, I mean triglyceride that is contained within a lipoprotein, even though it is measured as a total quantity without regard to which lipoprotein carries it in the blood.

Cholesterol's Exit

The body has two main processes by which to dispose of cholesterol. One is excretion of cholesterol as neutral sterols, and the second is conversion of cholesterol to bile salts. Both forms of cholesterol derivative are lost in the feces. That is, cholesterol is converted to bile salts that are secreted, along with neutral sterols, into the gallbladder and excreted via the biliary system into the upper small intestine when we eat a meal. Bile salts help in the digestion and absorption of the fat coming from the stomach contents as they enter the small intestine. When this process goes awry, gallstones may form. If too much cholesterol-derived sterols or salts build up in the gallbladder, excess cholesterol precipitates as gallstones.

The body recycles the bile salts via reabsorption (98–99%) by the intestine, so fecal loss (1–2%) of excess cholesterol via bile salts may not be efficient enough to keep cholesterol in check. When individuals eat too much cholesterol, the liver not only shuts down synthesis of more cholesterol by the body but, unfortunately, also reduces the number of LDL receptors on cells that could help remove cholesterol from the blood by pulling it into the liver for disposal via the bile. This shutdown of the removal process is a major problem with high dietary cholesterol intake. Lowering intake of dietary cholesterol helps increase the number of LDL receptors on cells, particularly liver cells, which increases the rate of removal of cholesterol from the blood. Therefore, not only does lowering dietary cholesterol reduce the influx of exogenous cholesterol, it will also help increase the rate of uptake of the cholesterol that is in the blood in the form of LDL particles. The movement of cholesterol through the bloodstream is closely linked with that of triglycerides.

Cholesterol Tends to Rise with Age

Many physicians consider total blood cholesterol under 200 mg/dl and triglycerides under 150 mg/dl to be desirable values for adults with no other risk factors, such as a previous heart attack or diabetes. Blood lipid values are not as well studied in children, but those given for adults are often followed for children as well. An elevation in both cholesterol and triglycerides is a common scenario for many people, so much so that it is often referred to as garden-variety hyperlipidemia because there are no clear genetic causes, diet may influence it, and it often gets worse with age and obesity. Genetic background of individuals, like age, is important; however, it is frequently not clear what genes are involved. In North America and Europe a common form of hypercholesterolemia, familial combined hyperlipidemia, is present in 10–15% of patients with myocardial infarction. The condition is characterized by an oversynthesis of VLDL and LDL, thus LDL cholesterol and triglycerides are often elevated together in the blood (Kane and Havel 2001). It has been associated with a variety of genetic variations, including alterations in the apoE genotype, variations in regulation of apoB expression, and lipoprotein lipase polymorphisms, along with other less well understood genetic variations.

Familial combined hyperlipidemia is clearly polygenic in nature. This is in stark contrast to the single-gene *(monogenic)* example of familial hypercholesterolemia (FH), which is caused by mutations in the low-density lipoprotein (LDL) receptor gene (Goldstein, Hobbs, and Brown, 2001). Patients with FH will have elevated cholesterol values all their lives, including childhood. Familial hypercholesterolemia patients who are heterozygous for this dominant disease trait are found in the general population at a rate of about 1 in 500, whereas familial combined hyperlipidemia is about 15 times more common.

Regardless of genetic heritage, aging effects are strong, especially for women as they go through menopause. The strongest risk factor for cardiovascular disease is age. Of course, age is like genetics: we can't do much about it. So let's look at a risk factor for cardiovascular disease that can be reduced, and that is elevated blood lipids. In general, premenopausal women under 50 who don't smoke tend to be more resistant than men to hyperlipidemia and cardiovascular disease. This may be at least partly due to the fact that premenopausal women who show this resistance also tend to collect excess adipose tissue in the posterior (buttocks), instead of the abdomen, as men do. Recall that excess fat in the buttocks is safer than excess fat in the belly because it is not associated so much with hyperlipidemia and insulin resistance.

Not only does the natural process of decreasing endogenous estrogen during menopause affect lipid metabolism, so does estrogen replacement therapy. That is, physicians find that women who are on oral estrogen, even for short-

Table 4.2. Classification of dyslipidemias

Dyslipidemia	Blood lipid characteristics	Diagnoses
Hypercholesterolemia	Increased LDL	Polygenic hypercholesterolemia; familial hypercholesterolemia; familial defective apolipoproteinemia
Combined hypercholesterolemia and hypertriglyceridemia	Increased VLDL and LDL	Familial combined hyperlipidemia or simple combined hyperlipidemia
	Increased chylomicron remnants and IDL	Often called type III hyperlipoproteinemia
	Increased chylomicrons and VLDL	Familial lipoprotein lipase deficiency
Hypertriglyceridemia	Increased VLDL	Familial or sporadic hypertriglyceridemia
Hypoalpha-lipoproteinemia	Low HDL	Associated with hypertriglyceridemia; heterozygous mutations in *ABCA1* or *APOA1*
Hypobeta-lipoproteinemia	Low LDL and VLDL	Familial truncated apolipoprotein B

Source: Summarized from Durrington 2003.

Note: ABCA1, gene for the ABCA1 transport protein required for reverse cholesterol transport via HDL; *APOA1*, gene for apolipoprotein A-I, a component of HDL; HDL, high-density lipoprotein; IDL, intermediate-density lipoprotein; LDL, low-density lipoprotein; VLDL, very low-density lipoprotein.

term relief of bad menopausal symptoms, tend to have elevated blood triglycerides, in contrast to those receiving transdermal estrogen via the estrogen
patch. The reason may be the amount of oral estrogen directly affecting liver
lipid metabolism as it is absorbed via the normal digestive process. In sum,
the common forms of fat-related diseases (hyperlipidemia or dyslipidemia)
are characterized by growing worse with aging, especially in postmenopausal
women. These diseases may follow familial patterns, like familial combined
hyperlipidemia, but most often a clear-cut genetic cause cannot be identified.
This is because disease processes like dyslipidemia result from the interaction
of multiple genes in combination with environmental and behavioral factors.
Dyslipidemia is very common.

Some patients have only elevated blood cholesterol concentrations or only
elevated triglyceride concentrations, and some have elevations in both (Gotto
1999; Durrington 2003). Certain patterns can be detected from observing
many patients over time (see Table 4.2). Many of the disorders described in
Table 4.2 are not clear-cut, single-gene disorders like FH. But some of the
single-gene disorders have characteristics similar to those that appear to be
caused by multiple genetic differences, along with diet and exercise effects.

In other words, some individuals with significantly elevated LDL cholesterol would be described as having hypercholesterolemia (Table 4.2), but they
do not have a genetic deficiency of LDL receptors. For example, some patients
have elevated LDL cholesterol along with hypothyroidism or chronic liver disease and have normal alleles for LDL receptor genes. Furthermore, hardly any-
body fits exactly into neat categories. There is the "textbook" case, and then
there are the "real" cases that must be fit into the best possible category, but
often not exactly.

A major point I want to get across is that genetics plays a role in the development *(pathogenesis)* of the more common varieties of hyperlipidemias. This
is especially so for combined hypercholesterolemia and hypertriglyceridemia,
which accounts for more than 85% of the cases of hyperlipidemia. The impact
of genetic makeup in most of these situations, however, is much less clear-cut
because multiple genes may be acting in a particular combination. Behavioral
and environmental factors (diet and exercise) also contribute to the net result
we see as hyperlipidemia, as well as to long-term consequences such as diabetes or cardiovascular disease.

It is important to appreciate the difficulty of figuring out the primary and
secondary causes of these diseases. Familial patterns are evident in the incidence and character of these diseases, but we cannot assume that the cause is

mostly in the "genes." Families—generation after generation, for better or worse—tend to eat similar foods and have similar exercise patterns, and these also have a major effect on the development of hyperlipidemia. Scientists in this area of medicine would like to figure out the exact set of factors, genetic and environmental, that cause disease. Then they might be able to develop preventive measures, new drugs, or even gene therapy in extreme cases to correct the problem. There are clearly people who are extremely prone to hyperlipidemia because of their genetic constitution, but scientists do not yet understand the genetic factors well enough to devise specific therapies. On the other hand, there are various other reasons (be it fast-food marketing, excess carbohydrates, decreases in physical activity due to increased television, computer games, etc.) for the rapidly increasing incidence of obesity, insulin resistance, hyperlipidemia, diabetes, and cardiovascular disease in the general population. Since our gene pools have not changed that much that fast, our environment and behavior must be having a major influence.

National Cholesterol Education Program

Since 1985 the National Heart, Lung, and Blood Institute (NHLBI) of the National Institutes of Health (NIH) has sponsored the National Cholesterol Education Program (NCEP). The goal of NCEP is to reduce coronary heart disease in the United States by reducing the number of Americans with high blood cholesterol. To that end expert panels have been assembled to develop guidelines for lowering cholesterol in patients, the most recent of which are the Adult Treatment Panel III (ATP III). This wealth of information is readily available on the website listed in Table 4.3. The guidelines, directed toward physicians treating patients with hypercholesterolemia, require that the physician take into account the full health characteristics of the patient, including various risk factors of heart disease, before making specific recommendations to the patient. Providing an overview of those issues is beyond the scope of this book, but see Table 4.3 for an outline of the ATP III guidelines for blood cholesterol concentrations.

In addition, at the NCEP website there is a calculator for estimating your risk of developing myocardial infarction and coronary death in the next ten years. At the website you enter the answers to the following queries: (1) age, (2) gender, (3) total cholesterol concentration, (4) HDL concentration, (5) smoking status, (6) systolic blood pressure (top number), and (7) medicines

Table 4.3.   Guidelines for interpreting cholesterol concentrations in adults, from the National Cholesterol Education Program

Concentration (mg/dl)	Classification
LDL cholesterol	
< 100	Optimal
100–129	Near optimal/above optimal
130–159	Borderline high
160–189	High
≥ 190	Very high
Total cholesterol	
< 200	Desirable
200–239	Borderline high
≥ 240	High
HDL cholesterol	
< 40	Low
≥ 60	High

Source: NCEP-ATP III guidelines (www.nhlbi.nih.gov/guidelines/cholesterol/atp3upd04.htm).

taken for high blood pressure. An immediate calculation of risk, based on equations developed from the Framingham Heart Study, is provided for you.

This chapter has focused on the various types of hyperlipidemia (disease characteristics are summarized in Table 4.2). Obviously, genetics, diet, and exercise can have major effects on the net body fat characteristics. These characteristics include the amount of body fat, as well as excessive blood cholesterol or triglycerides, and fatty change in liver and muscle, and they can influence the development of insulin resistance and nonalcoholic steatohepatitis (NASH). The Human Genome Project promises eventually to help in clinical medicine, as clinicians better understand these multifactorial disease traits like hyperlipidemia. Chapter 10 focuses on the clear-cut single-gene disorders of elevated cholesterol and triglycerides. In the next chapter I will move on to discuss another common accompaniment to hyperlipidemia, and that is development of insulin resistance and its expanded disease version, known as metabolic syndrome.

CHAPTER 5

Insulin Resistance and Metabolic Syndrome

In most cases it takes years or even decades to develop type 2 diabetes. The prelude to full-blown diabetes is insulin resistance, which occurs when the pancreas has to secrete more and more insulin to get the same effect of glucose uptake by the body. I believe, from current research findings of my own and from many others, that abnormal fatty acid metabolism is at the root of this problem. You will learn in this chapter about the characteristics of insulin resistance and associated disease problems like obesity, high blood pressure, risk for heart disease, and others. I also explain that there are at least three different names to a syndrome that is very common.

Insulin Resistance

Insulin is an extremely important hormone that regulates cellular metabolism and growth. Insulin is required for glucose influx into muscle and fat cells, among others. Insulin resistance is defined as the condition whereby the body's cells require more and more insulin to get the same effect of glucose uptake. Suppose an individual has normal insulin sensitivity with a blood glucose value of 140 mg/dl after a meal. If given 10 units of rapid-acting insulin, he or she will experience a drop in blood glucose within minutes to 85 mg/dl. Now let us suppose that the person is insulin resistant. After eating the same meal, he or she has a blood glucose value of >200 mg/dl and, if given the same 10 units of insulin, experiences no drop in blood glucose level at all. This is the functional definition of insulin resistance. It is this process occurring again and again over the years that eventually leads to overt diabetes: the pancreas eventually cannot keep up with making enough insulin to overcome this growing insulin resistance. Processes occurring within the pancreatic β-cells also appear to cause their eventual death, and that's when the insulin concentrations fall and diabetes occurs.

Liver, brain, and red blood cells do not require insulin action for uptake of blood glucose. Although insulin is not required by liver cells for glucose uptake, it regulates important functions in liver cells. One such process is the liver's production of glucose, called *gluconeogenesis*. Gluconeogenesis, which means "new glucose," is the process of synthesizing glucose from noncarbohydrate precursors, such as amino acids. Gluconeogenesis is needed when a person has not eaten for a few hours and blood glucose concentration is beginning to fall. As glucose storage as glycogen in the liver is reduced during fasting, blood glucose concentrations must be maintained if the person is to remain conscious. At that point gluconeogenesis normally begins to make glucose and the liver burns fatty acids as the required fuel in order to do it. The liver can then provide newly made glucose to help maintain blood glucose concentrations during the period of fasting. In contrast, in the fed state, insulin normally shuts down gluconeogenesis when blood glucose is already high. In fat cells, insulin is required to suppress the lipolysis of stored triglycerides and the resulting release of free fatty acids and glycerol. The problem in insulin-resistant states is that gluconeogenesis is not shut down and lipolysis, especially of visceral adipose tissue, is not suppressed. That is, the liver is making too much glucose and the visceral adipose tissue is releasing too many fatty acids flowing directly to the liver. Increasing glucose stimulates the pancreas to produce more and more insulin, and the vicious cycle known as insulin resistance begins. Normal mechanisms of regulation of insulin secretion are lost, and tissue response even to excess insulin is abnormal. The result is ever increasing blood glucose concentrations that in turn stimulate more insulin secretion.

Metabolic Syndrome

Insulin resistance is the centerpiece of a common syndrome originally described by Gerald Reaven of Stanford University as syndrome X (Reaven 1988; Reaven, Strom, and Fox 2000). In addition, it is also commonly referred to as insulin resistance syndrome or metabolic syndrome. I will refer to it as metabolic syndrome. Regardless of what it's called, this syndrome is a very common clinical pattern seen in patients who are on their way to developing diabetes and cardiovascular disease. It has been estimated that 24% of U.S. adults now have metabolic syndrome (Ford, Giles, and Dietz 2002). The common features include obesity, rising blood glucose concentrations, increased blood insulin concentrations *(hyperinsulinemia)*, increased blood triglyceride concentrations *(hypertriglyceridemia)*, increased small, dense LDL cholesterol (a potentially bad form of LDL cholesterol), decreased blood HDL concentrations, high blood pressure *(hypertension)* frequently accompanied by heart enlargement *(cardiac hypertrophy)*, and blood coagulation dysfunction. The diagnostic characteristics are shown in Table 5.1. A patient with this collection of metabolic abnormalities often is developing diabetes and cardiovascular disease.

Although obesity is common among patients with metabolic syndrome, not all obese people have it, and thin people can have the syndrome. Nevertheless, obesity is considered a risk factor for metabolic syndrome. The syndrome has a strong association with the development of heart disease, although the mechanisms linking the two remain controversial. Furthermore, many patients, if untreated, go on to develop type 2 diabetes.

Type 2 diabetes mellitus is also known as noninsulin-dependent diabetes.

Table 5.1.   Diagnostic criteria of metabolic syndrome

National Cholesterol Education Program	World Health Organization
ATP III guidelines require 3 or more factors to be present	Insulin resistance (detected by decreased glucose tolerance, or presence of type 2 diabetes) plus any two additional criteria
Abdominal obesity-waist circumference Men > 40 inches Women > 35 inches Blood triglycerides ≥ 150 mg/dl HDL cholesterol Men < 40 mg/dl Women < 50 mg/dl Blood pressure ≥130/≥85 mm Hg Fasting blood glucose ≥ 110 mg/dl	Obesity: BMI > 30 or waist/hip ratio > 0.9 men > 0.85 women Blood triglycerides ≥ 150 mg/dl HDL cholesterol Men < 35 mg/dl Women < 40 mg/dl Elevated blood pressure ≥ 140/90 or on blood pressure drugs Urinary albumin excretion rate > 20 μg/min; albumin/creatinine ratio > 30mg/g[a]

a. Presence of albumin in the urine is a common finding in insulin-resistant patients. Albumin loss in the urine may be expressed as an excretion rate or as the ratio of albumin to creatinine, a breakdown product of metabolism that is normally found in urine. See Ford, Giles, and Dietz (2002) for further information.

This is because type 2 patients do not tend to develop acute, life-threatening ketoacidosis if they do not receive insulin treatment. Type 2 patients, however, may take insulin for treatment. Chapter 6 describes the differences and similarities between type 1 and type 2 diabetes. Type 2 diabetes, the one that follows development of metabolic syndrome, most often develops in people over the age of 50 years. The typical patient is overweight to obese, sedentary, and frequently has a family history of type 2 diabetes. In fact, having a parent or a sibling with type 2 diabetes is the strongest risk factor, other than age, a person can have for developing diabetes, regardless of obesity or exercise. Typically, these folk go to their doctor and find out that their blood lipids and glucose concentrations are high.

Impaired fasting glucose (a prediabetic condition) is defined as having a fasting plasma glucose over 100 mg/dl but less than 126 mg/dl. Diabetes is now diagnosed by detecting a fasting plasma glucose concentration of 126 mg/dl or higher, a value set by an Expert Committee (2003) of the American Diabetes Association. In practice, diagnosis often involves finding this value on two occasions or finding a nonfasting blood glucose concentration of >200 mg/dl.

Type 2 diabetes does not develop overnight. It may take decades of increasing insulin resistance until the pancreatic β-cells cannot keep up with the body's increasing need for higher and higher insulin secretion, and then the blood glucose concentrations become abnormally high (Figure 5.1). Generally, by the time an individual is diabetic, insulin resistance is as bad as it is going to get. Developing diabetes is more a matter of how well the pancreatic β-cells can fight the uphill battle of insulin resistance. Unfortunately, with the growing number of children developing type 2 diabetes, the disease more often requires only years, rather than decades, to develop.

The Starting Point

How metabolic syndrome starts is a fairly controversial issue. The process is complicated, yet it clearly involves a combination of a patient's genetic background, sex, diet, and exercise habits. Part of the controversy has to do with what happens first. What are the causes and what are the effects? As an example, some believe insulin resistance causes obesity, whereas others believe obesity causes insulin resistance. A common underlying factor is the abnormal buildup of fat. This may be due to excessive fat in the adipose tissue stores, excessive fat buildup in the liver and muscle cells, or even having too little adipose tissue available for proper storage of fat in the body (this occurs in lipodystrophy, as I mentioned in Chapter 1). Another important factor is the location of the excess adipose tissue in the patient's body. Is the predominant adipose storage of body fat "in the butt or in the gut"? Clinically, does the patient have the shape of a "pear" or the shape of an "apple" (Matsuzawa 1997)? As discussed earlier, adipose tissue buildup in the butt area is considered subcutaneous fat, and it is harder to get free fatty acids released from this fat during fasting, whereas beer-belly fat is visceral fat, and it is readily available for easy buildup, breakdown, and release of free fatty acids into the blood. Excess visceral fat, which is more sensitive to hormonal signals for fat breakdown, seems to be a constant source of fatty acids that build up in the blood. The take-away message is that the pear shape may be unsightly but healthwise more desirable than the apple shape. That is, subcutaneous fat is somewhat "safer" to carry around than the visceral gut fat.

As you can imagine, the complex combination of variables—genetics, sex, diet, and exercise—affects the processes involved in developing elevated fatty acids in the blood. I believe a high concentration of free fatty acids in the blood is the key factor in developing insulin resistance. In other words, if a low concentration can be maintained, the patient can avoid most if not all of the

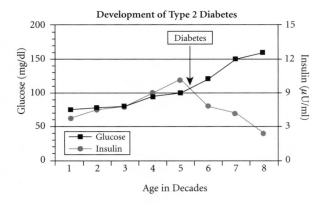

Figure 5.1. The body may be able to respond to rising fasting blood glucose concentrations with increasing insulin production for decades, but eventually the pancreas may not keep up with the increasing demand. For the person whose glucose and insulin concentrations are presented in this idealized graph, that point was reached between 50 and 60 years of age. The evaluation of insulin and glucose levels is complex because the amount of insulin in the blood at any one time is determined by several factors: insulin secretion, which occurs in two phases in response to glucose load, clearance of insulin by the liver, degree of insulin resistance present, and other variables.

other problems of metabolic syndrome, including the development of insulin resistance and eventually type 2 diabetes mellitus. Sumo wrestlers are certainly obese, yet as long as they exercise they remain insulin sensitive. Surprisingly, in addition to exercise, eating a diet relatively high in unsaturated fatty acids but low in total calories may actually help lower blood levels of fatty acids; I will explain this heretical statement in the Chapter 13. Yes, a "relatively" high-fat diet of "healthy" fats, but low in total calories, may be more healthful than a low-fat, high-carbohydrate diet consisting of starch and sugar.

Relationship between Free Fatty Acids and Glucose

Understanding the fluxes of both fatty acids and glucose is crucial to understanding the molecular mechanisms of metabolic disease. It is my own view, however, that rising concentrations of fatty acids in the blood are the *cause*, and rising levels of insulin in the blood are the *effect*, of metabolic syndrome. A complex interaction exists between the amount of free fatty acids in the blood and the amount of triglyceride building up in visceral adipose tissue, liver, and muscle. There is growing interest in the possible direct effects of fatty acids on the pancreatic β-cells that produce and secrete insulin. Additionally, a growing body of data strongly indicates that an excessive buildup of triglyceride in muscle and liver is a major indicator that insulin resistance is occurring. That is, when tissues not intended to store fat, such as liver and muscle, become overrun with fatty acids and cannot "burn" them completely, then these nonadipose tissues store them as triglycerides. This is not healthy. Using advanced imaging techniques of patients' muscles and liver, scientists have found that quite a lot of triglyceride can be stored there, especially in those patients with the most severe insulin resistance and with elevated free fatty acids in the blood. It appears, then, that the elevation of triglycerides in tissues is the body's way of compensating for the buildup of fatty acids in the blood, which delivers the excess fatty acids to the cells. Fatty acids are toxic to cells and are quickly converted to acyl coenzyme A (acyl-CoA) molecules, which are either oxidized for energy or used to synthesize triglyceride. In some tissues, like liver, cells may also synthesize even more fatty acids in excess of demand, which may end up as surplus triglyceride. Investigators can actually see this triglyceride by using magnetic imaging techniques in insulin-resistant patients.

Gerald Shulman and colleagues have shown that the real culprit here is likely the buildup of excess acyl-CoA concentrations in cells (Shulman 2000).

They found that the excess in acyl-CoA can develop from different underlying events, including aging and the subsequent loss of mitochondrial function, as well as from a genetic predisposition for reduced mitochondrial function found in offspring of patients with type 2 diabetes (Petersen et al. 2003, 2004). For whatever reason, reduced mitochondrial function, including β-oxidation of fatty acids, increases the potential for a buildup of acyl-CoA and development of insulin resistance in those cells. Thus, when excess fatty acids in the blood enter cells and are converted to acyl-CoA, they may end up as stored triglyceride. Apparently, not all acyl-CoAs are being converted to triglyceride and they are certainly not being burned away, so acyl-CoA concentrations may also become excessive. Excessive acyl-CoA appears to interfere with a critical step when cells are activated by insulin.

The insulin receptor activates a whole cascade of signaling events, which include the activation of proteins that are known as insulin receptor substrate (IRS) molecules, IRS-1 and IRS-2. The activated IRS-1 in turn activates the enzyme phosphatidylinositol-3 (PI-3) kinase. PI-3 kinase is key for many of the expected actions of insulin on cells, especially muscle cells (Shulman, 2000). This includes stimulating glucose transport into cells from the blood in order to lower blood glucose. Cells activated by insulin should have an increased expression of the enzymes required for the breakdown of glucose for energy production via glycolysis and glucose oxidation. If glucose is metabolized normally—that is, if it is broken down into its component molecules such as pyruvate, which is then further oxidized to produce energy—there is no backup in the process. During insulin resistance, when glucose cannot get into the cell for this metabolism to occur, the glucose concentrations in the blood will rise.

Meanwhile, insulin-resistant cells in the liver are not reducing the production of glucose, which only makes the whole problem of high blood glucose worse. This excess glucose stimulates more insulin release, and the vicious cycle continues. There are many other failed steps in this cycle, and these are most easily detectable when they cause rising blood glucose concentrations and increased insulin values—in other words, "insulin resistance." Therefore, the consistent characteristics of insulin resistance include elevated fatty acids in the blood and tissue storage of excessive triglycerides. There is universal agreement on those characteristics. The flip side, as you will see, is that conditions that lower the concentration of fatty acids in blood markedly improve insulin sensitivity.

Reducing Fat Reduces Insulin Resistance

Although the mechanisms that result in insulin resistance may look fairly straightforward, the story is much more complicated than I have described in this brief summary. It's important to realize that many genetic variables, along with dietary and behavioral effects, contribute to the net development of insulin resistance. I think you can already see what has to happen to fix the problem: decrease the fat in the blood. Lowering fatty acid concentrations will reduce the buildup of intracellular acyl-CoA in tissue, which in turn allows PI-3 kinase to work properly. In this way, the insulin resistance process can be reversed. That is, with PI-3 kinase working properly, glucose uptake and glucose metabolism will be restored in the tissues, especially in muscle. This process increases the "insulin sensitivity" of the cells.

To reduce the fat burden, two things must happen. First, increasing the amount of aerobic exercise will increase the burning of fat. This will help a great deal to clear the whole body of excess fat, including tissues and the blood. The second step is to eat a diet that will decrease free fatty acids and fat storage. This sounds easy but is in itself a complicated issue (explored in Chapter 13). No one will argue the benefits of increasing dietary fiber, especially soluble fiber, and also simply eating fewer calories. There are good reasons to reduce intake of total calories, but it may also be beneficial to pay attention to the type of foods eaten. Substituting some healthy fat (polyunsaturated and monounsaturated fats) in the diet in place of excessive sugar and starch helps many people to reduce their blood triglycerides and presumably the fatty acids in blood and tissue. Dr. Reaven, who originally described syndrome X, recommends a ratio of protein calories (15%), fat calories (polyunsaturated and monounsaturated fats, 30–35%, and limited saturated fat, 5–10%), and carbohydrate calories (45%) (Reaven, Strom, and Fox 2000). This approach remains a controversial topic in human nutrition and metabolism research.

Nonalcoholic Steatohepatitis (NASH)

Another common disorder in patients with hyperlipidemia, obesity, and insulin resistance is steatohepatitis, the accumulation of fat in the liver plus inflammation. This is a separate disease from any of the viral hepatitis diseases. It seems to be a metabolically induced liver problem, but scientists are just now putting together clues about this disease. It is not to be confused with alcoholic cirrhosis of the liver, characterized by inflammation, hepatocyte cell death *(necrosis)*, and fibrosis of the liver.

With the increase in the numbers of people with obesity, insulin resistance, and hyperlipidemia, there has been an increase also in nonalcoholic fatty liver disease (NAFLD), a commonly used broader term that includes NASH (Browning and Horton 2004). NASH can appear similar to liver disease caused by chronic alcohol intoxication, but it occurs in people who are not alcoholics, though the most severe cases can end up with liver cirrhosis. The reason this disease is so alarming is that approximately 50% of obese people have fatty liver most of the time. It is estimated that 10% of those patients will develop some form of NASH. This is a disease affecting millions of people that is clearly associated with all of the common lipid problems previously discussed, especially hyperlipidemias. Scientists have not yet figured out all of the factors that trigger this liver disease process in some people and not others. Excess fat storage in the liver appears to be the most common underlying factor. With fatty liver being the first "hit," there also appears to be some second "hit" required that induces NASH (Browning and Horton 2004). The second "hit" remains unknown in people, although recent studies in animal models are providing important clues to pursue.

To summarize, the commonly occurring metabolic syndrome and its cornerstone insulin resistance may eventually lead to the development of type 2 diabetes, cardiovascular disease, and other chronic disorders. This disease process is frequently aggravated by obesity. A gross imbalance in fatty acid metabolism appears to be an underlying mechanism in the development of this disease; that is, too many fatty acids and not enough fatty acid oxidation. The approach to therapy includes lifestyle changes such as reduced calorie intake and increased activity level. Both help reverse these processes in most people by reducing the overall body load of stored fat. Lifestyle changes are sometimes not enough, so drugs may be used to reverse insulin resistance by the same mechanism, reducing fatty acids in the blood to clear the tissues of excess fat. This will be explored in much more detail in the next chapter, on diabetes. Some people simply have an unfortunate combination of genetics that makes control of insulin resistance challenging; however, even they can often help themselves by eating less and exercising more.

CHAPTER 6

Type 1 and Type 2 Diabetes

Patients with diabetes mellitus are often considered as one large group experiencing a single disease; however, this is not the case. There are two major groups of patients with diabetes: 90–95% of patients are type 2 and the rest type 1. Although both types of diabetes are characterized by elevated blood glucose concentrations, the diseases develop from two entirely different sets of circumstances. Type 1, or what was called insulin-dependent diabetes, is an autoimmune disease in which the immune system damages the pancreatic β-cells, resulting in profound insulin deficiency. In contrast, type 2 diabetes results from years to decades of insulin resistance. Insulin resistance is a condition in which glucose metabolism, which begins with activation of cells by the hormone insulin, becomes less and less effective, and the pancreas has to produce more and more insulin. Type 2 diabetes occurs when the pancreas cannot keep up. Type 1 patients are often slim and prone to potentially fatal ketoacidosis, whereas type 2 patients are often obese and rarely have problems with ketoacidosis. In the later stages of both types of diabetes, many disease processes affect the cardiovascular system, nervous system, and eyes.

Different Causes of Diabetes

Diabetes mellitus (DM) literally means the excessive production of "sweet urine." In Latin *mellis* means "honey." Thus historically, the focus of diabetes has been on the sugar component of the disease; in this chapter I intend to convince you we must pay a lot of attention to the fat side as well.

There are several types of diabetes, the main ones being types 1 and 2 diabetes mellitus. The different types have a range of underlying disease factors that involve genetic predisposition for autoimmune disease or obesity and rare mutations of genes controlling the synthesis of enzymes, transcription factors, and receptors that directly affect metabolism (Taylor 1995). The hallmark of diabetes is abnormally high blood glucose concentrations, resulting in glucose loss by the kidney with glucose found in the urine. Elevated blood glucose concentrations develop because many cells in the body, especially those in the muscle mass, are not being activated by insulin to begin the process of actively taking up glucose for energy generation. In type 1 diabetes mellitus (DM1), the problem is the lack of insulin, but in type 2 diabetes mellitus (DM2) the initial problem is the inadequate cellular response to insulin.

Glucose tolerance is usually associated with the body's response to a glucose load, such as a glucose tolerance test. Glucose intolerance reflects β-cell dysfunction and insulin resistance resulting in a prolonged disappearance of glucose from the blood when challenged. Glucose intolerance is a signal event. Once the body fails to process glucose properly, a sequence of events is put in motion that can lead to progressively more debilitating illness. Among the possible consequences are cardiovascular disease, including both macrovascular and microvascular lesions, kidney disease, often eventually leading to dialysis, disease of the extremities, such as problems in the feet, nervous system disease, and disease of the eye, including the lens and the retina.

Approximately 90–95% of diabetic patients in the United States have type 2, or "noninsulin-dependent," diabetes (DM2), whereas the remaining 5–10% of patients have "insulin-dependent" DM1. The American Diabetes Association recommends the use of the terms type 1 and type 2 diabetes rather than making reference to insulin. In general, DM1 patients must have insulin therapy in order to survive, so that form was called insulin-dependent DM, whereas DM2 patients are only sometimes treated with insulin, and their disease is not acutely life threatening.

Since blood glucose is the hallmark test of the disease, many people do not realize that diabetes, of both types, is as much a disease of fat metabolism as it is a disease of glucose metabolism. The late Denis McGarry published a review in *Science* magazine in the early 1990s in which he very eloquently and effectively raised awareness of this fact (McGarry 1992). I believe diabetes, especially DM2, is primarily a disease affecting fat metabolism and that high blood glucose happens to be a good clinical marker to monitor. Certainly, elevated blood glucose causes many problems as well. In addition, both types of DM share some of the long-term complications, including cardiovascular disease, circulation problems in the feet, eye disease, neuropathy, and kidney disease. Nevertheless, in many ways, these two types of diabetes are quite different, at least in the early stages. In the later stages the differences are less clear. Eventually patients with DM2 may become insulin deficient, require insulin therapy, and develop the same chronic diseases as those associated with DM1.

Type 1 Diabetes

Type 1 diabetes results from profound insulin deficiency. It occurs most frequently in children, although it can happen in adults also. That is, many adult DM1 patients had the disease when they were children. Clinically, it seems to happen suddenly, almost overnight in some cases. Patients may notice that they are urinating very frequently, including many times during the night, and it may go on for a few weeks. Some may even develop an acute gastrointestinal upset with vomiting. Others may experience a sudden and unusual weight loss accompanied by increased hunger and thirst.

DM1 is most often caused by an autoimmune disease against the pancreatic β-cells that normally produce and secrete insulin when blood glucose concentrations are high. This process of immune injury to the pancreas may begin months before the patient has any signs of disease. Any disease process that causes death of pancreatic β-cells will produce DM1, but autoimmune disease is the most common cause.

The pancreas has two major functions (Table 6.1). The exocrine portion of the pancreas produces digestive enzymes that are secreted into the upper small intestine (duodenum). The endocrine portion produces, among other things, insulin and glucagon and releases them into the bloodstream. Insulin

Table 6.1. Functions of the pancreas

Exocrine portion	Endocrine portion (islets of Langerhans)

Acinar cells secrete digestive enzymes
    Protein digestive enzymes: trypsin, chymotrypsin,
      elastase, carboxypeptidase
    Carbohydrate digestive enzymes: α-amylase
    Fat digestive enzymes: pancreatic lipase, colipase,
      and phospholipase A$_2$
	α-cells produce glucagon
	β-cells produce insulin
	
	δ-cells produce somatostatin

is needed in times of nutritional plenty, like after a meal, to promote for glucose uptake by tissues, stimulate the storage of glucose as glycogen, and shut down the oxidation of fatty acids while promoting for fatty acid and triglyceride synthesis. Insulin is synthesized by the β-cells of the pancreatic islets, which are patches of cells that are distinctly different from the exocrine pancreatic gland cells. The islets have β-cells for producing insulin and α-cells for producing glucagon. Glucagon, the hormone that has effects opposite those of insulin, is active when insulin is low. Glucagon is at the highest blood concentrations, and has the greatest effect, during a fasting period, when blood glucose is dropping and alternative fuel sources for the body are needed, such as fatty acid oxidation (burning fat). Glucagon is used for glycogen breakdown, increases glucose synthesis by the liver (gluconeogenesis), and stimulates fatty acid oxidation. *Glycogen* is the form in which the body stores glucose in the tissues: a long chain of sugars linked end-to-end. So although they both come from the pancreatic islet cells, insulin and glucagon have essentially opposing actions.

Patients with DM1 develop an immune reaction against their own pancreatic β-cells. The β-cells are destroyed by the infiltration of lymphocytes in an inflammatory reaction. As a result, the cells lose virtually all of their capacity to produce insulin, and everything that is supposed to occur when insulin is needed doesn't happen. In fact, glucose metabolism seems to be further aggravated by the continued production of glucagon with no counterbalance of normal insulin action. Here's what happens.

Once the insulin receptor stops mediating glucose transport, the cells' ability to take up glucose is compromised. Fatty acid oxidation increases, and body stores of fat are being broken down to supply the excessive demand for fatty acid oxidation. Many untreated patients with DM1 lose body fat as a result of this process and therefore appear lean. The liver is making excessive glucose because insulin is not halting its production. So, in effect, not only has the system lost the "brakes" to this process by the lack of insulin, but it now has an uncontrolled "accelerator" with glucagon action unopposed. As a consequence, the patient has very high blood glucose (>500 mg/dl; normal should be <95 mg/dl), is urinating a lot because glucose is being lost in the urine, and is becoming dehydrated because of the excess water loss. The kidney filters glucose from the blood but normally reabsorbs it as the filtrate is processed within the kidney. When blood glucose reaches around 180 mg/dl blood concentration, the kidney cannot reabsorb glucose quickly enough, and that is when glucose begins to "spill over" into the urine.

The other key feature of DM1 is the dangerous development of ketoacidosis. In Chapter 9, I will explain the normal process of producing ketone bodies as an alternative fuel when fasting. Ketone bodies are the extended products of fatty acid oxidation. In Chapter 10 I will discuss the problems children with inherited diseases of fatty acid oxidation deficiency have because of their dangerous inability to produce ketone bodies when challenged by fasting. In DM1, the opposite problem exists: fatty acid oxidation and ketone body synthesis are out of normal control because of the insulin deficiency and the relative glucagon excess. This is the life-threatening stage of acute DM1.

My research team in the 1990s used a mouse model of DM1, the *nonobese diabetic* (NOD) mouse, for studies (Kurtz et al. 2000). In a series of experiments with these mice, we showed that the expression of fatty acid oxidation enzymes rose in mice that developed the acute mouse form of diabetes. This of course supports the idea that ketoacidosis results from excessive fatty acid oxidation when the insulin brake is absent. In mice and in people, this disease course happens because the insulin-producing cells have been destroyed by the body's own immune system.

Autoimmunity against β-Cells

Scientists still don't know what molecular events trigger the body's immune attack on the β-cells, but they do have a few promising leads. Increasingly, a genetic risk factor appears to be the culprit. See Eisenbarth, Ziegler, and Colman (1994) for an excellent overview of the pathogenesis of human DM 1, which I have summarized here.

Many DM1 patients have inherited a particular allele combination of genes that code for human lymphocyte antigens (HLA). Lymphocytes are the specialized white blood cells that are essential for immune reactions against infections. When things go wrong, however, lymphocytes can also attack body tissues. The pancreatic islets are being attacked as if they were an infection or a foreign tissue (as if the body were rejecting a mismatched transplant).

The first step in this autoimmune process is the inheritance of particular alleles of HLA genes. After this first "hit," the second appears to be a viral infection of some sort. Several viruses have been implicated, but none has been proven to be the culprit. Sometime after the viral infection, the patient begins developing an autoimmune inflammatory reaction against the body's own pancreatic β-cells and soon (within days or weeks) develops the life-threatening insulin deficiency. Virtually all DM1 patients have antibodies against their pancreatic islet cells. So, DM1 results from a profound insulin deficiency caused by β-cell loss. DM1 patients are usually insulin sensitive, and if regulated insulin secretion occurred in their bodies, all processes would function normally.

Insulin Resistance and Type 2 Diabetes

Insulin resistance occurs when it takes more and more insulin, secreted by the β-cells of the pancreas, to keep blood glucose concentrations in the normal range, although the glucose concentrations tend to creep up as this process progresses. At some point after years of insulin resistance, the β-cells go from a dysfunctional oversecretion of insulin to a process of cell failure. As a result of this change, the need for large amounts of insulin is no longer met, and blood glucose concentrations rise above the diagnostic level (at fasting, 126 mg/dl). There is now a "relative" insulin deficiency but not an absolute insulin deficiency, as occurs in DM1. Once a patient's blood glucose concentrations pass beyond the accepted "normal" threshold, the clinician makes a diagnosis of DM2. So insulin resistance will lead up to the onset of DM2 and it will continue after DM2 has been reached. In other words, virtually all DM2 patients are insulin resistant, but not all insulin-resistant patients have DM2.

DM2, the much more common form of diabetes, is often diagnosed after a decades-long process of increasing insulin resistance; it is rarely the result of a relatively sudden insulin deficiency. The development of insulin resistance involves a general backup of fatty acid oxidation, or an ongoing process of excess of fatty acid synthesis. The net effect is that fatty acids are increasing in the blood and in tissues such that there is a buildup of unmetabolized fatty acids in the form of triglyceride. If one were to continue cutting wood for a fireplace that is only burning a small amount, the wood supply will pile up. The solution is to reduce the rate of chopping wood or to burn more of it in a larger fireplace. This is, in effect, the problem faced by a person with insulin resistance and DM2: too much extra energy backed up.

This slowing down of fatty acid oxidation is relative. Fatty acid oxidation is not profoundly deficient—the problem for patients with inborn errors of fatty acid oxidation (Chapter 10). Given the fat load, from either the diet or endogenous synthesis, the amount of fat burning is deficient for the situation. My research team tested this hypothesis directly by evaluating fatty acid oxidation gene expression measures of liver in the *obese* mutant mouse model (Brix et al. 2002). These mice are three times heavier than normal mice because they are deficient in the hormone leptin (see Chapter 1). We expected to see an abnormally low level of expression of enzymes needed for fatty acid oxidation in the livers from these mice. Overall, we found normal levels of these enzymes, but their livers were loaded with triglyceride. The *obese* mice are also insulin resistant throughout most of their life. When we evaluated their oxidation of whole-body fat, in addition to specific measures in the liver, we found no significant differences from the normal controls. Therefore, given their fat load, these mice were relatively deficient in fatty acid oxidation.

In contrast to the DM1 patient, whose fatty acid oxidation is out of control and who is experiencing dangerously excessive ketogenesis and potential acidosis, the DM2 patient usually is not undergoing ketoacidosis. (More details about ketoacidosis are in Chapter 9.) This is also the case in the insulin-resistant patient who is gradually converting to DM2. The two types of DM share high blood glucose concentrations, but they are at the opposite ends of the spectrum as far as fatty acid metabolism is concerned. The type 2 DM patient is often obese and has an inappropriately low rate of fat burning, with excessive fat building up in many tissues; the type 1 DM patient is often lean as a result of excessive fat burning. Even type 1 diabetes patients can put on extra weight once they are treated with insulin. When type 2 patients reach a condition of severe β-cell failure, they may be insulin deficient and appear clinically as equivalent to a type 1 diabetes patient. In Table 6.2 the features of DM1 and DM2 are compared.

Therapy for the Different Types of Diabetes

Physicians and other clinicians use different treatment approaches and drug regimes for patients with DM1 and DM2. DM1 is almost exclusively treated with insulin injections. Patients require daily blood glucose monitoring and insulin injections according to the blood glucose concentrations, along with careful dietary control of sugar and fat intake. A major problem in treating DM1 is the need to balance the timing of insulin injection and food intake: the patient may have more trouble with insulin-induced low blood glucose (*hypoglycemia*) than hyperglycemia. When experiencing hypoglycemia, the patient has to have a piece of hard candy or a sugar-containing soda to raise the blood glucose concentration to avoid passing out. Insulin must be given by injection or some other non-oral means because it is a protein and, like any protein, will be digested if taken by mouth. So far, there is no substitute for insulin therapy in the DM1 patient. There are various ways of administering insulin, such as an insulin pump, but there simply is no other way around the profound insulin deficiency that occurs in this disease. Researchers are at-

Table 6.2. Common features of type 1 and type 2 diabetes mellitus

Clinical Features	DM1	DM2
Etiology	Genetics (HLA) and environment (viral infection?)	Genetics (multiple genes not identified) and environment (calorie intake/activity level)
Blood glucose concentrations	180–500 mg/dl	110–130 mg/dl
Body type	Lean	Obese
Ketones in urine	Positive	Negative
Glucose in urine	Positive	Negative
Treatment for high glucose	Insulin	Insulin sensitizers; oral hypoglycemic agents; insulin

tempting islet-cell transplants in the hope of restoring the patient's own ability to synthesize insulin.

Treatment of DM2 patients may first be directed at reducing blood concentrations of glucose and fatty acids, as well as reducing the triglyceride load in the blood, muscle, and liver so that increased insulin sensitivity may reverse the process. Patients are often aggressively treated for hyperlipidemia, as described in Chapter 4. The most commonly used drugs for these patients are of four basic types: (1) sulfonylureas, which increase insulin output by the already overworked pancreatic β-cells, are prescribed to lower the blood glucose concentrations, (2) biguanides, when used alone, act to reduce fatty acids and increase insulin sensitivity without causing hypoglycemia, (3) α-glucosidase inhibitors reduce the intestinal digestion of sucrose, starches, and maltose, resulting in reduced blood glucose concentrations after eating, and (4) thiazolidinediones (TZDs), also known as glitazones, increase insulin sensitivity by decreasing the blood concentrations of free fatty acids. The TZDs may also reduce the inflammatory state found in insulin-resistant patients. See Table 6.3 for examples of the currently available drugs for treating DM2. All of these

Table 6.3. Generic and brand names of type 2 diabetes drugs

Class of drugs / Function	Generic and brand names
Sulfonylureas Promote increased β-cell secretion of insulin	acetohexamide (Dymelor) chlorpropamide (Diabinese) glimepiride (Amaryl) glipizide (Glucotrol) glyburide (DiaBeta, Glynase PresTab, or Micronase) tolazamide (Tolinase) tolbutamide (Orinase)
Biguanides Increase sensitivity of cells to insulin; decrease hepatic glucose output	metformin (Glucaphage)
α-Glucosidase inhibitors Reduce digestion of sugars and starches; lower blood glucose concentrations after eating	acarbose (Precose)
Thiazolidinediones Increase sensitivity of cells to insulin by reducing blood fatty acid concentration; anti-inflammatory agent	rosiglitazone (Avandia) pioglitazone (Actos)

drugs have strengths and weaknesses, but those issues are beyond the scope of this chapter. In addition, many DM2 patients must also receive insulin therapy. Eventually, if this process of overworking the β-cells is not relieved by improving insulin sensitivity, the β-cells appear to fail, and the patient may develop an insulin deficiency and other symptoms that occur in DM1 patients.

Hemoglobin A_{1c} for Monitoring Diabetes

Measurements of glycosylated hemoglobin, hemoglobin-A_{1c} (HbA$_{1c}$), are used to monitor both types of diabetes (see Figure 6.1). This is the measurement of a normally small percentage of total hemoglobin molecules that have a glucose molecule attached. On average, red blood cells that carry hemoglobin in the blood circulate about 120 days. Glucose enters red blood cells without any need of insulin action. Over time, the amount of glucose inside the red blood cell, where the hemoglobin is located, equilibrates with whatever the blood glucose concentration is on the outside in the blood plasma. So individuals

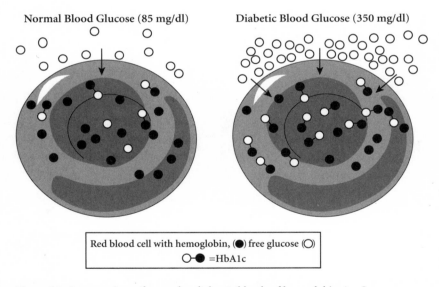

Figure 6.1. A comparison of normal and elevated levels of hemoglobin-A_{1c}. In a person with hyperglycemia, blood glucose concentration is high and more glucose molecules move into red blood cells (illustrated at right). Once inside the blood cell, the free glucose attaches to a hemoglobin to form HbA$_{1c}$. The percent of total hemoglobin having an attached glucose changes slowly, so it is a good measure of long-term control of blood glucose.

with normal blood glucose concentrations—let's say a value of 85 mg/dl—will have a certain percentage of red cell hemoglobin molecules with a glucose molecule attached. The glucose is attached to hemoglobin in the red cell by an irreversible, nonenzymatic attachment process. Normally, around 3–4% of the total amount of hemoglobin will be glycosylated (HbA$_{1c}$). If the blood glucose concentration is high over the lifespan of the red cell—for example, in a poorly controlled diabetic patient—then the concentration of glucose in red cells will be high, the reaction of glucose attaching to the hemoglobin will occur more often, and the percentage of HbA$_{1c}$ will be higher, 7–9%. The usual goal for treatment is to keep HbA$_{1c}$ below 7%.

This measurement reflects the average glucose concentration in the blood over a few weeks. The typical blood glucose measurement is simply the concentration at the instant when the blood sample was drawn. Patients who have been skipping medicines or eating too much sugar could simply take their insulin right before going to the doctor. The blood glucose concentration may look fine by this measurement, when in fact it has been out of control for several weeks. The real value of HbA$_{1c}$ measurements is that they reflect the longer-term average blood glucose—and the patient can't cheat on them.

Long-Term Complications of Diabetes

Several disease processes may be set in motion by diabetes, and that is why using tools (like measuring HbA$_{1c}$) for maintaining the best possible glucose control is so important. Blood lipid control is likewise essential and as important as glucose control. Long-term complications of uncontrolled diabetes include cardiovascular disease, decreased circulation to the feet, increased risk for heart attacks, kidney disease, eye disease, and peripheral neuropathy, and an increased susceptibility to infections. Diabetes of both types is much more than a disease of high blood glucose concentrations. Successful management of these diseases requires careful monitoring and long-term control of both glucose and fat metabolism. Demands are made on both the patient and the clinician, because therapy involves much more than simply taking medicines—it requires matching the diet and activity level with the medicines.

Type 1 diabetes is caused initially by an autoimmune disease or some other process that destroys the pancreatic β-cells, resulting in profound insulin deficiency. Type 2 diabetes appears to be the outcome of a decades-long process of increasing insulin resistance such that the pancreas eventually cannot keep up with the demand for insulin production. Eventually the β-cells fail to produce the extra insulin required to keep blood glucose in the normal range, and the patient develops frank diabetes. This process of insulin resistance and β-cell failure can end up as an insulin-deficiency disease if it is not halted or reversed as soon as possible. Both diseases can have similar long-term consequences, such as cardiovascular disease, neuropathy, kidney disease, and eye disease.

Since excess fat is a crucial component of the development of insulin resistance and important in the long-term disease processes of diabetes, in the next section of the book I will present more detailed explanations of the processes in the body that are involved in the intake, synthesis, and storage of fat and the reverse process of fat oxidation. If a balance is not reached between fat accumulation and fat burning, obesity and insulin resistance will develop.

PART II

Dynamics of Fat Metabolism

CHAPTER 7

The Energy Equation

This chapter serves as an introduction to the idea of energy balance. From this basic perspective, diseases of excess fat are fairly simple to understand: too many fatty acids in the body and not enough fatty acid burning. What leads up to this imbalance, however, is extremely complicated and a tremendous challenge to change. As is the goal of this entire book, I want you to understand how risky excess fat is to overall health, and how much better off people are if they can shed some of their excess fat or, better yet, prevent it altogether. The good news is that if calorie intake matches calorie expenditure, there is no way to gain weight as fat. We can work both sides of this energy equation. The concept of balance is simple, even though the reality of maintaining it is a major challenge.

Eating Behavior Is a Key Factor

Virtually all of the genetically obese mouse mutants are hyperphagic, which is a fancy way of saying they eat a lot. Their extreme obesity is caused by mutations in the genes that regulate feeding behavior. Research shows that it is food intake that is the more critical factor, not the ability to burn fat, although fat metabolism may also be involved.

Research suggests that at an individual level, eating behavior drives human obesity, and our genetics may play a significant role in that behavior. My own research team studies mice with genetic deficiencies of fat oxidation, but obesity is not a major feature in these mutants. We must recognize that the quantity of food people eat is a critical factor and, unfortunately, that exercising off excess weight is a terribly inefficient method of weight control. As shown in Table 7.1, it is probably easier for most people to reduce their food intake 300 calories (by giving up a dessert per day, for example) than to burn up 300 calories (by walking 3 miles per hour for an hour every day). I will explain in some detail in the upcoming chapter on exercise. Please do not misunderstand my point here: Overall activity level, including exercise, is an important part of a healthy lifestyle, but for most people it is easier to eat fewer calories than to burn off the extra calories with exercise in order to lose body fat.

Another important distinction to understand is that body fat mass is what should be reduced, not body weight per se. It is not healthy to lose weight by losing muscle mass. As a result of increased exercise, muscle mass could increase at the same time that body fat is being reduced, resulting in no change, or even a rise, in body weight. A cubic centimeter of muscle is significantly heavier than the same volume of fat. Leanness is the goal, not a number on a scale.

Exercising and Activity Level Is the Other Key

Energy expenditure or output is the other side of this critical equation of body fat and diseases of excess fat. Exercise can help with initial body fat loss; however, exercise seems to be more effective in maintaining leanness. Exercise helps reduce many disease processes, such as insulin resistance, independent of a decrease in body fat. Reducing excess body fat helps even more. Even without weight loss, people who get their muscles working and burning excess

Table 7.1. Metabolic effects of calorie reduction, increased activity, or both combined

Change in diet and exercise	Calorie loss per year	Fat loss per year
Calorie intake reduced by 300 calories per day; activity level remains constant	300 cal x 365 days = 109,500 cal / yr	31.3 lb
Calorie intake remains constant; daily activity increased by 1 hr walk (3 mph)	319 cal x 365 days = 116,435 cal / yr	33.3 lb
Calorie intake reduced and activity increased	225, 935 cal / yr	64.6 lb

a. Note that dietary "calories" equal kilocalories of energy.
b. Assume that 3,500 cal = 1 lb of fat.

fat will increase their insulin sensitivity. Overall reduction of blood concentrations of fatty acids leads to improved insulin sensitivity and reduction of triglycerides in the blood. Exercise facilitates the lowering of fatty acid concentrations.

Net Energy Balance

As far as calories are concerned, what goes in must be balanced by what goes out (Rosenbaum, Leibel, and Hirsch 1997). If excess fat is already present, then there must be a reduction of what goes in and an increase of what goes out. A calorie is a calorie is a calorie. There are no foods that counteract the calorie content of other foods. There may be ways in which people take in food calories that reduce feelings of hunger, resulting in a corresponding reduction in calorie intake, but a calorie is a calorie. Calories will be either burned or stored. What many people do not realize is the gradual additive nature of weight gain as fat over time. Rosenbaum, Leibel, and Hirsch (1997) point out as an example that if calorie intake exceeds expenditure by only 2% daily for a year, the result is a gain of approximately five pounds for that year. Eating an extra 100 calories per day will add over 10 pounds of extra fat per year. Reducing calorie intake and increasing activity level will decrease body fat, and reducing body fat will reduce the disease processes associated with excess fat.

The clinical presentation of obesity is socially and emotionally far more complex than the energy-balance equation. Relearning the eating behaviors of a lifetime, adjusting daily habits to increase physical activity, learning not to resort to food for comfort or to relieve boredom—all these are part of the challenge. Many physicians who see desperate, morbidly obese patients resorting to gastric bypass can attest to the fact that not all cases of obesity can be cured by dieting. Initial weight loss is not unusual, and relatively easy, follow-

Table 7.2. Metabolic goals confront real world challenges

Metabolic goals	Social challenges
Calorie intake matched with energy expenditure to remain lean	Cultural/family influences on learned eating behaviors
	Food advertising
Low body burden of fatty acids	Processed foods with added sugar, unhealthy fats, and salt
Normal insulin sensitivity	Sedentary workplaces
	Suburbs designed for cars and not people

ing a new dieting regimen, but keeping the weight off is another matter. In addition to learned behaviors, there are genes that affect metabolic rate, muscle types, lipoprotein characteristics, exercise endurance, and many other influences on a person's ability to overcome obesity. The current epidemic of obesity is a complex problem (Table 7.2), one whose solution may include public health measures, government policy toward health care, school and city design, advertising—all of which are beyond the scope of discussion here. The chapters that follow focus on the individual, but in Part IV I will return to some of these larger issues.

CHAPTER 8

Making and Storing Fat

Fatty acids are the building blocks of the lipid molecules known as triglycerides. Triglycerides constitute the predominant form of fat in adipose tissues and in food. In addition to being derived from the dietary triglycerides, fatty acids may also be synthesized by the body from sugar. This chapter will track dietary fats and examine the role that chylomicrons and VLDLs play in transporting triglyceride for use or storage. The liver is critically important as the "Grand Central Station" controlling the fatty acid and triglyceride fluxes in the body. A major conductor regulating these processes is insulin.

Origins of Triglyceride

As noted in Chapter 3, fatty acids are essential components for building triglycerides and phospholipids. These fatty acids either are made by the body or come from the diet. Now let's follow the intake of triglycerides and fatty acids from the diet into the tissues, as we did for cholesterol in Chapter 4. In Western society, and increasingly elsewhere around the world, dietary fat comes from animal sources (meat, poultry, fish, dairy products, and eggs), from certain fat-rich plant foods (primarily nuts and seeds), and from the oils we add during food preparation. Most of this dietary fat is in the form of triglycerides. As the triglycerides enter the stomach and make their way into the upper small intestine, stomach acids, bile salts, and digestive enzymes known as *lipases* begin breaking them down into fatty acids and glycerol (Figure 8.1). Digestive lipases are manufactured in the pancreas and bile salts come, via the gallbladder, from the liver. Once the fatty acids are free, they enter the cells lining the small intestine, where they are reassembled as triglycerides and formed into chylomicrons. Chylomicrons eventually end up in the blood via the lymphatic system draining the intestines.

Once in the bloodstream, the chylomicrons along the way can exchange triglyceride for cholesterol esters from HDL. Further on their trek, another enzyme, *lipoprotein lipase*—found in the capillary beds of muscle, heart, adipose tissue, and other nonliver tissues—will strip the triglyceride in the chylomicron of its fatty acids. As the chylomicron is stripped of triglyceride and

The journey of fat after eating:

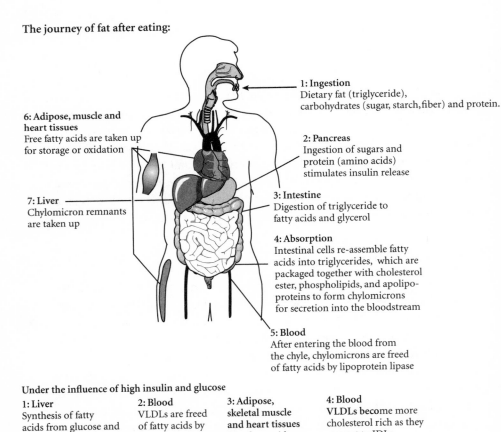

6: Adipose, muscle and heart tissues
Free fatty acids are taken up for storage or oxidation

7: Liver
Chylomicron remnants are taken up

1: Ingestion
Dietary fat (triglyceride), carbohydrates (sugar, starch, fiber) and protein.

2: Pancreas
Ingestion of sugars and protein (amino acids) stimulates insulin release

3: Intestine
Digestion of triglyceride to fatty acids and glycerol

4: Absorption
Intestinal cells re-assemble fatty acids into triglycerides, which are packaged together with cholesterol ester, phospholipids, and apolipoproteins to form chylomicrons for secretion into the bloodstream

5: Blood
After entering the blood from the chyle, chylomicrons are freed of fatty acids by lipoprotein lipase

Under the influence of high insulin and glucose

1: Liver	2: Blood	3: Adipose, skeletal muscle and heart tissues	4: Blood
Synthesis of fatty acids from glucose and secretion of triglyceride as VLDL	VLDLs are freed of fatty acids by lipoprotein lipase at tissues	Free fatty acids are taken up for storage or oxidation	VLDLs become more cholesterol rich as they convert to IDLs and then LDLs

Figure 8.1. The fate of dietary fats and their components following a meal.

apolipoprotein C (apoC), it arrives at the liver for uptake as a chylomicron remnant. More than 90% of the triglyceride originally found in the chylomicron will be broken down by lipoprotein lipase into free fatty acids, which will be deposited around the body before the chylomicron remnant finally ends up at the liver.

The "Grand Central Station" for Fatty Acid and Triglyceride Flux

After an individual has eaten, when blood glucose concentration increases, the pancreas increases insulin secretion and reduces its output of glucagon. Insulin is the principal manager of the "Grand Central Station"—the liver—at this point. In contrast, the production and secretion of glucagon are nil at this point, but glucagon will take over when times are lean, such as a fasting period. Insulin activates cells for the synthesis and storage of energy in the forms of glycogen (sugar) and triglycerides (fat), as well as synthesis of protein. Since the liver receives the insulin signal for energy storage when it is operating with a plentiful glucose supply (after a meal), its functions are to store the incoming fatty acids or send them on for storage elsewhere, like adipose tissue. The first stop for any incoming fatty acids will be in the formation of triglyceride again. Any synthesis of fatty acids that occurs from carbohydrate sources, like glucose, will also be assembled into triglycerides. Free fatty acids are toxic to cells, so when they enter the cell they are bound to intracellular fatty acid binding proteins and quickly converted to acyl coenzyme A (acyl-CoA). In this form the fatty acid substrate is ready to be oxidized by mitochondria for energy generation or used to form triglycerides. Since insulin concentration is high, fatty acid oxidation is turned off, and the predominant fate of these fatty acids will be to build triglycerides.

The liver cells now begin assembling VLDL particles for export of the fatty acids originally derived from the food. In an individual with normal metabolism, there should be no substantial buildup of triglyceride in the liver during this period. When the store of triglyceride in the liver becomes excessive, the condition is known as fatty liver *(hepatosteatosis)*. As I described earlier, hepatosteatosis is very common in people with obesity and diabetes mellitus. It is basically a backlog of "fat" trains trying to leave the station. Not every one can get out and the station becomes overcrowded. The only way to clear the station is to reduce the incoming supply of passengers (fatty acids), increase the number of trains (VLDLs) leaving, or transfer part of the fat load to another mode of clearance, such as fatty acid oxidation. In this analogy, fatty acids are the passengers, sitting three to a seat (triglyceride), in a train car (VLDL). The triglyceride is repeatedly broken down into fatty acids and then reassembled into triglycerides throughout this process, because only the single passengers are going to enter muscle or adipose cells as they leave their seats on the train cars.

The VLDLs, rich in triglyceride, are now headed out of the liver into the bloodstream to supply fatty acids to the rest of the body. Some of the VLDL triglyceride will end up in the capillary beds of muscle tissue, ready to provide fatty acids for energy. The rest will enter adipose tissue as fatty acids that are converted yet again into a triglyceride and then stored away. The VLDLs will be acted upon by lipoprotein lipase in the capillary beds of muscle and adipose tissue to generate free fatty acids. Once inside the cell, the fatty acids are converted to acyl-CoA and metabolized for energy production by the muscle. Additionally, adipose tissue will take them up for regeneration into triglyceride and for fat storage. As mentioned earlier, as the VLDL loses triglyceride it becomes an intermediate-density lipoprotein (IDL). With the further loss of apoE and triglyceride, IDLs become LDLs, which are rich in cholesterol. The remaining lipoprotein particles are involved mostly in cholesterol transport, which was discussed in Chapter 4. That is the end of the journey for the majority of triglyceride originating from lipoproteins generated by the liver. It is certainly not the end of the line for the fatty acids and triglycerides that originate from the diet.

Destinations of Fatty Acids and Triglycerides

Fatty acids are deposited at several sites as they are released from triglyceride being carried by either chylomicrons or VLDLs. Some are left at the muscles, including heart muscle, and will be used to produce energy through mitochondrial fatty acid oxidation. VLDL triglycerides are predominantly deposited as fatty acids in the muscle rather than the adipose tissue. Most of the fatty acids that reach adipose tissue are brought by chylomicrons for storage and future use. These are quickly resynthesized into triglyceride for storage. Other fatty acids are left at the liver, where they are either metabolized for energy or stored as triglyceride, but many are probably incorporated into VLDL for export out of the liver.

When triglycerides reach a cell, they are either stored or burned or broken down by oxidation carried out by cellular organelles, mitochondria or peroxisomes. Since insulin is high and the body is in storage mode, the balance is in favor of storage. The only way to eliminate the stored triglyceride is to use it as energy. Of course here is the problem. If it is not used for expending energy, it remains for an extended stay as stored fat. The bulk of this stored fat will be in adipose tissue, but it can also build up in liver and muscle. And there is more to come! So far I have described the fate of the fat that comes in through the diet and have not yet brought up the ugly fact that the body can also synthesize fat from excess carbohydrates.

The Body Turns Sugar into Fat

After a person eats, insulin concentration is high, and it promotes for energy storage. Starches and other carbohydrates will be broken down to simple sugars like glucose by digestion for absorption. Glucose stimulates insulin secretion. Insulin will also promote for storage of glucose, in the form of glycogen, in the liver, muscle, and other tissues. Glycogen has many storage limitations. It attracts water, which takes up cellular space, and it is heavier than stored fat. Although glycogen is an important source of quick energy needed to maintain blood glucose upon fasting, and thus keeps us from passing out from hypoglycemia, it is not an efficient way to store energy for long-term needs. Fat storage is much more efficient. First, fat does not attract water; it repels it, so it is more compact to store. Second, fat has a higher calorie density per gram than sugar or protein. Fat has 9.3 kcal/gram, whereas sugar has 4.1 kcal/gram and protein has 4.0 kcal/gram. So there is approximately twice the energy stored per gram of fat stored and no water "baggage."

One explanation for easy, early weight loss on virtually any diet is that if someone reduces calorie intake and draws on the glycogen stores, the loss of the associated water is quickly reflected by the scale. Overnight changes in body weight are almost always due to changes in body water status: the underlying cause may be changes in glycogen content, changes in salt intake, drugs that promote for water loss such as diuretics, vigorous exercise with lots of sweating, or conditions such as kidney disease. No one is going to gain or lose a few pounds of fat or muscle overnight, although weight may change that much. In Table 8.1, I have outlined the advantages and disadvantages of glycogen and fat storage.

Given the tissue distribution and deposition of digested fat, you may already begin to see ways it starts building up more than we would want: in the liver as hepatosteatosis, in adipose tissue as excess fat storage, and even in muscle as myosteatosis. After the body has stored away the glucose as glyco-

Table 8.1. Advantages and disadvantages of glycogen vs. fat storage of energy

Advantages	Disadvantages
Glycogen storage	
Ready source of quick energy	Attracts water and is a heavy and bulky storage form of energy
Maintains adequate blood glucose concentrations between meals	Has limited capacity for storage; not useful as long-term energy source
Fat storage	
Has twice the calorie density of glucose	If stored in the wrong places, tends to promote for insulin resistance
No water attraction, so it is a more compact and lighter form of energy storage	Not as readily used up; tends to build up over time with excess calorie intake and reduced energy expenditure

gen, where possible and with the volume limitations described, the liver may start making more fatty acids from the excess glucose. These fatty acids can then make their way to adipose tissue storage via the triglycerides in VLDL particles. Human adipose tissue has a low capacity for fatty acid synthesis, unlike adipose tissue of rodents. In earlier periods of human history, during the leaner times of hunting and gathering, this ability to store energy was essential for survival. Nowadays, however, with mega-sized fast food on every corner, such highly efficient storage is not needed. In fact, it becomes a liability for health. Since the insulin released after a meal promotes energy storage, what happens when excess glucose remains even after the glycogen stores in liver and muscle have been replenished? Unfortunately, it can turn into fat.

Glucose contributes to the synthesis of triglyceride in two important ways. First, it provides the two carbon units required for synthesis of fatty acids via malonyl-CoA. Second, it provides the starting material or substrate for generating the glycerol used to connect together the three fatty acids in a complete triglyceride.

Fatty acid synthesis was worked out in the late 1940s and later by Konrad Bloch, whom we met previously in the section on cholesterol synthesis, David Rittenberg, Salih Wakil, Feodor Lynen, and Roy Vagelos. Fatty acids are produced during times of plenty and when insulin is high, because insulin stimulates the activity of a key enzyme, acetyl-CoA carboxylase (ACC). ACC produces malonyl-CoA, which is crucial for two reasons. One is that malonyl-CoA is the building block of fatty acids. Its net contribution is the addition of two carbon units to the growing fatty acids. The other is that it reduces mitochondrial fatty acid oxidation. Malonyl-CoA is a potent inhibitor of carnitine palmitoyltransferase-1, the enzymatic "gatekeeper" of mitochondrial fatty acid oxidation. These dual effects of malonyl-CoA are complementary: if the goal for the moment is to store energy as fat, burning of fat should be turned off.

The other component needed not only for generation of malonyl-CoA by ACC but also for fatty acid synthesis is acetyl-CoA. Acetyl-CoA is the end product of both glucose oxidation and fatty acid oxidation, but as I described, fatty acid oxidation is drastically reduced when insulin levels are high. Insulin promotes the uptake of glucose by cells. This intracellular glucose is used for quick energy generation and longer-term energy storage processes, including synthesis of glycogen and triglyceride. Therefore, when acetyl-CoA is generated during times of plenty (i.e., high glucose and insulin), its primary source is glucose. Besides, why would the body break down fat while it simultaneously builds fat?

Malonyl-CoA, a three-carbon molecule, is made from acetyl-CoA by addition of a carbon dioxide molecule. As shown in Figure 8.2, the way fatty acid synthesis works is this: the cell starts off with both an acetyl-CoA and a

High Insulin and Glucose Promote for Fatty Acid Synthesis

High Insulin

$$\text{Glucose} \xrightarrow[\text{Glycerol}]{\text{Glycolysis}} \rightarrow \rightarrow \text{Acetyl-CoA} \xrightarrow{\text{Acetyl-CoA Carboxylase (ACC)}} \text{Malonyl-CoA}$$

Fatty Acid Synthesis

Step 1 $\quad C_2$-acetyl-CoA + C_3-malonyl-CoA = C_4-acyl-CoA(fatty acid) + CO_2

Round 2 $\quad C_4$-acyl-CoA + malonyl-CoA = C_6-acyl-CoA(fatty acid) + CO_2

3 $\quad\quad\ \, C_6$-acyl-CoA + malonyl-CoA = C_8-fatty acid + CO_2

4 $\quad\quad\ \, C_8$-acyl-CoA + malonyl-CoA = C_{10}-fatty acid + CO_2

5 $\quad\quad\ \, C_{10}$-acyl-CoA + malonyl-CoA = C_{12}-fatty acid + CO_2

6 $\quad\quad\ \, C_{12}$-acyl-CoA + malonyl-CoA = C_{14}-fatty acid + CO_2

7 $\quad\quad\ \, C_{14}$-acyl-CoA + malonyl-CoA = C_{16}-fatty acid (palmitate) + CO_2

Figure 8.2. The contribution of glucose as substrate for fatty acid synthesis via generation of malonyl-CoA. Malonyl-CoA provides a two-carbon addition to acyl-CoA during each round of fatty acid synthesis. Ultimately, the saturated C_{16} fatty acid, palmitate, is most often formed.

malonyl-CoA. A single carbon is lost as carbon dioxide (CO_2) in the process of combining the acetyl-CoA (C_2) and the malonyl-CoA (C_3). After one "round" of fatty acid synthesis catalyzed by the complex enzyme fatty acid synthase (Wakil 1989), the nascent fatty acid is four carbons long. Adding the malonyl-CoA units (C_3), originally derived from glucose, along with losing a carbon dioxide each round for six more rounds, lengthens this short fatty acid into one 16 carbons long. This is the saturated fatty acid known as palmitate (C_{16}). Mammalian cells produce fatty acids 16 carbons long only by the malonyl-CoA addition method. In the resulting fatty acid there are no double bonds—therefore, it is saturated. Making longer-chain fatty acids with double bonds requires separate enzymatic pathways for elongation and desaturation. Mammalian cells cannot produce the double bonds required to make the essential fatty acids. In Table 8.2 I have summarized the main points of fat synthesis from glucose.

Table sugar (sucrose, a glucose attached to a fructose) is broken down to the individual components of free glucose and free fructose. At the risk of redundancy, I want to emphasize here that sugar intake via its glucose component promotes for insulin secretion, which in turn promotes for fatty acid synthesis and reduced fatty acid oxidation. Fructose does not stimulate insulin secretion, nor does it require insulin for uptake by many cells, and it has a different but important impact on metabolism. Fructose is more rapidly metabolized by the liver than glucose, allowing it to facilitate fatty acid synthesis and increase the triglyceride load and VLDL production by the liver, as described earlier. The commonly used sweetener high-fructose corn syrup is over 50% fructose, and many believe is an important contributor to development of obesity and insulin resistance. Although fructose may be highly concentrated in fruits and fruit drinks, in excess it is as much a health risk as any excess sugar; perhaps, because it is more readily turned into fat than sucrose, in some ways it is even more potent than sucrose. In Table 8.3 I have outlined the key

Table 8.2. Contributions of glucose to triglyceride synthesis

1. Glucose metabolism generates acetyl-CoA, which is turned into malonyl-CoA.
2. Malonyl-CoA is the source of the two carbon units (C_2) that are connected together to build a fatty acid.
3. Glucose is also metabolized into glycerol, which is then used to connect three fatty acids into a triglyceride (3 fatty acids + 1 glycerol = 1 triglyceride).

Table 8.3. Insulin's role in fat storage

---

1. Insulin promotes for glucose uptake by tissues, followed by glycogen synthesis and glycolysis.
2. Insulin promotes for synthesis of glycerol and acetyl-CoA from glucose via glycolysis.
3. Insulin activates acetyl-CoA carboxylase, which produces malonyl-CoA.
4. Malonyl-CoA:
   a. Is the building block of fatty acid synthesis, which promotes for triglyceride synthesis.
   b. Inhibits fatty acid oxidation.
5. Insulin directly down-regulates fatty acid oxidation by mitochondria.

Overall, when insulin and glucose levels are both high, conditions are favorable for triglyceride synthesis and fat storage.

---

features of insulin's role in promoting fat storage. It is true, in other words, that a spoonful of sugar can end up as fat.

This chapter explored the building of triglycerides from fatty acids and how these lipids are transported around the body, as well as how they can be synthesized from sugar. Obviously, if the buildup and the breakdown of these lipids are out of balance, with the scales tipping toward the storage side, the potential exists for developing obesity and its related diseases. In the next chapter I will review the other side of this balancing act: the process of fatty acid oxidation.

CHAPTER 9

Burning Fat in the Cell

The body gets rid of stored fat when triglycerides are broken down into free fatty acids and glycerol and "burned" via mitochondrial fatty acid oxidation. This is an essential process during fasting or starvation and gives rise to ketone bodies. In some diabetic patients, excessive fatty acid oxidation and ketone body synthesis may occur, and the buildup of ketones can be very dangerous. Exercise promotes for fat oxidation, and the process by which that occurs is described. Specific dietary fats and drugs can also influence this process and lower blood lipids.

In the last chapter I reviewed the synthesis of fatty acids and storage of energy from a meal in the forms of fat and glycogen—that is, how fat enters the tissues of the body. I continue now with the process by which this energy, especially from fat, is expended—or where fat goes.

Destination of Stored Fat

A few hours after eating a meal, a healthy individual should have had his or her postprandial blood glucose peak combined with a secretion of insulin in response. After the major fluxes of lipid from the intestine and the liver have decreased, any temporary buildup of triglyceride in tissues, such as liver and muscle, should be cleared. The flux of fat from the liver—made of lipids derived from chylomicrons and lipids subsequently bundled in VLDL—will slow down: several hours after the end of a meal, the "rush hour" for fat and sugar entering the body's metabolism has ended. Also, as insulin begins to fall, endogenous synthesis of new fat slows down.

If no major energy expenditure occurs, such as exercise, the body still is slowly "burning," or oxidizing, these energy-containing nutrients to maintain normal body processes. That is, even when individuals are not exercising, their bodies are consuming a fair amount of energy just to keep the cells functioning. This is known as resting energy expenditure or resting metabolic rate. Basal metabolic rate is another term you may hear about, but it is very difficult to measure because the subject must remain inactive for a long period of time in thermoneutral conditions after a designated period since eating, and meet other conditions that are extremely difficult to reproduce. A tremendous amount of energy in the form of adenosine triphosphate (ATP) is required to maintain the salt, or electrolyte, balance between the inside and outside of even resting cells. The brain alone uses a lot of energy to maintain consciousness.

When blood glucose begins to drop below a comfortable set point, hunger pangs begin. Let's say that a person has decided to fast. This is when, short of exercise, the body begins to use that stored fat beyond just maintaining the body's homeostasis. Exercise, of course, also burns fat, but we'll get to that in Chapter 14. In Figures 9.1A and 9.1B I have contrasted the extreme metabolic events that occur in a sedentary individual after eating versus those occurring in a fasted athlete. It demonstrates how fat builds up in the first and is burned in the second.

Low blood glucose is a major trigger for the body to begin using backup energy mechanisms. When it starts falling because the diet-derived sugar has been used up and the glycogen that was stored in the liver is being depleted, something must happen or blood glucose concentrations will drop too low and the person will pass out. So a major goal of glucose homeostasis is to maintain consciousness. The way this is done is either to burn alternative fuels, like fat, in order to spare the glucose or to make new glucose from non-sugar sources by gluconeogenesis. Some tissues—such as heart and skeletal muscle, the so-called type I or slow-twitch skeletal muscle known for its oxidative metabolism—use fatty acid oxidation as their major fuel source most of the time. In contrast, the nervous system tends to be very dependent on glucose metabolism most of the time. Cells that can oxidize both glucose and fatty acids, like hepatocytes, will switch to fatty acid oxidation. This switch happens not only to save glucose for the brain, but also because gluconeo-

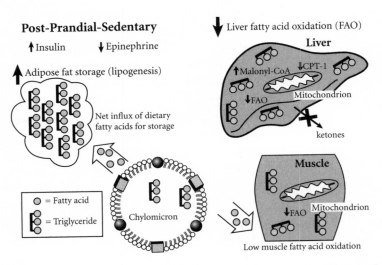

Figure 9.1A. Steps and conditions that lead to fat synthesis and storage. In this example, a sedentary person has just eaten a meal. The body is dominated by signals that promote for fat storage (high insulin) and there are few to no signals (low epinephrine) to promote for fat burning. Fat coming in from the diet via chylomicrons will be used for storage (in adipose tissues) or deposited in muscle for potential burning. In an insulin-resistant individual, excess fat will build up in liver and muscle.

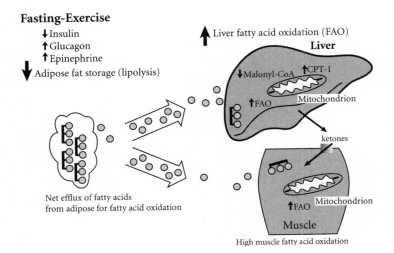

Figure 9.1B. A different set of conditions leads to fat burning in an active athlete who is fasting. In such a person insulin is low but glucagon and epinephrine levels are high, both of which promote fat burning. Fatty acids are released from adipose tissue and travel to liver and muscle, where they are targeted for further oxidation.

genesis is an energy-consuming process that must be fueled by oxidizing fatty acids in the liver.

Additionally, ketone bodies are produced by the liver as a by-product of fatty acid oxidation. Ketone bodies are synthesized and put into the bloodstream because they are used for energy by many tissues that would in times of plenty use glucose. Again the goal here is to spare glucose, and fatty acid oxidation allows this to occur. As the levels of insulin decline, the concentration of malonyl-CoA in the cells decreases, and some cell types (for example, hepatocytes) that had been busy making fatty acids are now reassigned to burn them instead. Whereas insulin was the hormone promoting for glucose and fat storage, glucagon, whose production is now rising, promotes for the opposite. Manufactured in the adrenal gland, epinephrine is responsible for, among other functions, spurring our "fight or flight" response. Thus epinephrine, with some actions like glucagon's, also puts the body into an energy-releasing mode. I have contrasted the different hormonal conditions and metabolic events of fed and fasting states in Table 9.1.

Fatty Acid "Burning"

By now, most of any triglyceride remaining after the meal has probably been oxidized by many cells, other than adipose tissue cells, which happened to store it temporarily. At this point the body will begin to burn the fat stored in the adipose tissue. Epinephrine, along with other lipolytic hormones, will promote for the breakdown of stored triglycerides by lipolysis. One of these (Table 9.2), because it is activated by epinephrine and other lipolytic hormones, is known as hormone-sensitive lipase. Again, insulin is the counterbalance because hormone-sensitive lipase is rapidly turned off when insulin is present

Table 9.1. Hormone actions in fed and fasted states

Fed state	Fasting state
Insulin	Glucagon
	Epinephrine/norepinephrine
1. Promotes for glucose storage (glycogen) and fat storage (triglyceride)	1. Promotes breakdown of glycogen
2. Promotes for reduced fatty acid breakdown from triglyceride (lipolysis)	2. Promotes for lipolysis
3. Reduces capacity for fatty acid oxidation	3. Promotes for fatty acid oxidation and ketone body synthesis

Table 9.2. Summary of lipase function

Lipase	Location of action	Function
Digestive lipase	Produced by exocrine pancreas and secreted into intestine for digestion	Break down triglycerides from food
Lipoprotein lipase	Found in capillaries of tissues other than liver, such as adipose or muscle cells	Break down triglycerides from lipoproteins
Hormone-sensitive lipase	Adipocytes	Break down triglycerides stored in cells

and the body is in storage mode. Hormone-sensitive lipase is different from the lipoprotein lipase discussed earlier. Recall that lipoprotein lipase is found in the capillaries of the adipose tissue along with other nonliver tissues. It works to free up fatty acids from the triglyceride in lipoproteins arriving to deliver fatty acids to these cells (for example, in adipocytes) for their conversion into triglyceride storage. Meanwhile, in counterbalance, hormone-sensitive lipase is waiting inside the adipocytes, ready to cleave triglycerides into free fatty acids and glycerol when activated by the lipolytic hormones.

Another hormone-activated protein that facilitates hormone-sensitive lipase activity for lipolysis is perilipin. During lipolysis, the fatty acids proceed in the direction going out of the cell toward the blood. Because fatty acids are not very water soluble, they bind to the blood protein *albumin.* Since they are bound to albumin temporarily, in loose bonds, they are known in this state as free fatty acids (FFAs) and also sometimes clinically as nonesterified fatty acids (NEFA).

The predominant lipolytic hormones in human beings are epinephrine from the adrenal glands or norepinephrine from the sympathetic nervous system. These lipolytic signals appear to work best when the stress hormone glucocorticoid and thyroid hormone are also present.

Once in the blood, free fatty acids are shuttled by albumin to tissues that can oxidize them and release their energy to do work in various organ systems. The major tissues that oxidize fatty acids are liver, heart, kidney, muscle, and brown adipose tissue. The liver is central to this process, the Grand Central Station of fatty acid metabolism. Brain tissue has very limited capacity for fatty acid oxidation and is more efficient at using the fatty acid oxidation by-product, ketone bodies. The type of adipose tissue that is most active at oxidizing fatty acids is the brown adipose tissue. Brown fat is found predominantly in babies; it is loaded with mitochondria capable of fatty acid oxidation and is important for heat generation by a process known as nonshivering thermogenesis.

First let's consider the liver, since it is central to many metabolic processes, especially during fasting (short-term, voluntary, relatively low emotional stress) or starvation (long-term, usually happenning in a body that is malnourished, high stress). During periods of lipolysis, hepatocytes will be bathed in blood carrying the fatty acid–loaded albumin. The fatty acids are unloaded at the hepatocytes and transported into the cell by fatty acid transport mechanisms. The fatty acids are then bound to proteins inside the cell. The free fatty acids will be converted to fatty acid derivatives, acyl-CoA, by the enzyme acyl-CoA synthetase. With coenzyme A (CoA) added to their ends, free fatty acids become the active form ready for further metabolism by the cell.

Most fatty acids found in the diet are long-chain fatty acids, with 16–18 carbons in a line (C_{16} to C_{18}). The human body synthesizes primarily C_{16} palmitate fatty acid, but it can also produce fatty acids with longer chains that are desaturated, such as the monounsaturated oleate ($C_{18:1}$). The fatty acids first stored in the adipose tissue and subsequently freed up for transport to the liver may reflect the dietary sources of fatty acid without much modification. Since most vegetable oils and meats have C_{16} to C_{18} fatty acids, those are the ones now presented to the hepatocyte for further metabolism.

Liver Action on Fatty Acids during Fasting or Starvation

You had to work late at the office, and now you are stuck in traffic, 90 minutes after you usually eat dinner and 6 hours since your lunch. Your stomach is growling. Your liver will be burning fatty acids by mitochondrial fatty acid oxidation to preserve glucose supplies until dietary carbohydrates arrive again. It does this by two major functions normally inhibited by insulin. Your liver receives glucagon and other signals to burn fat to provide the energy needed for glucose production via gluconeogenesis to maintain vital systems and consciousness. Lipids cannot be turned directly into glucose, but the energy from fat burning is used to convert the by-products of glucose catabolism, such as lactate and pyruvate, along with degraded protein components from muscle, known as glucogenic amino acids, into glucose. At the same time, the liver cells are making ketone bodies as an alternative energy source until glucose is once more plentiful. Ketone bodies are produced because muscle and several other tissues can use ketone bodies for energy, thus sparing glucose. Ketone bodies are made from the major product of fatty acid oxidation, acetyl-CoA.

The Process of Mitochondrial Fatty Acid Oxidation

Mitochondrial fatty acid oxidation is key to energy production, especially during periods of fasting. Medical geneticists and pediatricians know this because, unfortunately, babies with genetic deficiencies in fatty acid oxidation may not survive fasting (see Chapter 10). The process of fatty acid oxidation was elucidated by the work of several investigators starting at the turn of the twentieth century: Franz Knoop, Luis F. Leloir, J. M. Munoz, Albert L. Lehninger, Eugene P. Kennedy, Feodor Lynen, David E. Green, Severo Ochoa, Irving B. Fritz, and others. Greville and Tubbs (1968) published a very readable review of the discoveries leading to our present-day understanding of fatty acid oxidation.

Carnitine palmitoyltransferase-1 (CPT-1), the "gatekeeper" of mitochondrial fatty acid oxidation, was inhibited after eating because the high insulin levels promoted for production of malonyl-CoA, a potent inhibitor of CPT-1 action. Now, during fasting, everything is reversed: insulin is low, glucagon is high, and malonyl-CoA is very low. The previously inhibited CPT-1 is now used to bring fatty acids into the mitochondria for oxidation. The fatty acids coming into the hepatocytes from the blood are the substrate. Long-chain fatty acids cannot simply diffuse across the mitochondrial membrane but must be assisted by CPT-1 and other enzymes. CPT-1 functions to convert acyl-CoA into a new fatty acid derivative, acylcarnitine. Carnitine is a small molecule that, when it replaces the CoA on the fatty acids, makes the fatty acid capable of being transported through the double membrane surrounding the mitochondrion. CPT-1 action specifically replaces the CoA added to the fatty acid as it entered the cell with a carnitine to help it "slip" through the mitochondrial membranes. Another enzyme, carnitine-acylcarnitine translocase, then pushes the acylcarnitine on through these membranes. When the acylcarnitine makes it inside the mitochondrion, a final enzyme, carnitine palmitoyltransferase-2 (CPT-2), swaps the carnitine for another CoA, thereby reforming acyl-CoA.

The transported fatty acid, in the form acyl-CoA, is now inside the mitochondrion, in the innermost space known as the mitochondrial *matrix*. It is now ready for the actual oxidation process. Shown in Figure 9.2 is an overview of how fatty acid oxidation is stimulated when glucagon is high and at the same time insulin and malonyl-CoA concentrations are low. In contrast, elevated concentrations of malonyl-CoA, which form when insulin is high, inhibit fatty acid oxidation at the carnitine palmitoyltransferase-1 step (Figure 9.2—Step A).

This oxidation process is known as β-oxidation because it occurs at two-carbon intervals on the original fatty acid molecule, which is now in the form of acyl-CoA (Figures 9.3 and 9.4). β-Oxidation occurs at the second carbon from the end (COOH end) (Chapter 2, Figure 2.2), or the β carbon, in the chain. The goal of this process is to produce an energy-rich, two-carbon molecule known as acetyl-CoA.

As you will notice throughout these chapters, acetyl-CoA is the common

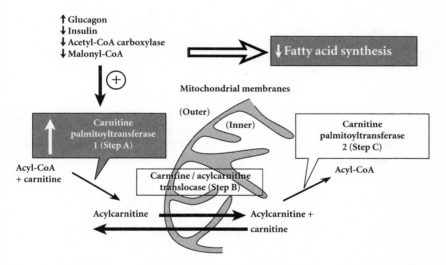

Figure 9.2. In the fasting state, high glucagon and low insulin levels activate fatty acid oxidation, which requires the enzyme carnitine palmitoyltransferase-1. CPT-1 is the gatekeeper of fatty acid oxidation. When it is inhibited following ingestion of food, fatty acid oxidation is low because the transport of fatty acid substrate into the mitochondrial matrix is reduced. After a period of fasting, however, the insulin-mediated brakes come off and fatty acid oxidation is stimulated. Fatty acids, in acyl-CoA form, must be converted into acylcarnitines, via the action of CPT-1, in order to be transported across the mitochondrial membranes (Step A). The next enzyme, carnitine-acylcarnitine translocase, moves the acylcarnitine across the mitochondrial membranes (Step B). Inside the mitochondrion, carnitine palmitoyltransferase-2 converts the acylcarnitine back into an acyl-CoA and carnitine (Step C). The carnitine shuttles back to the outside to be reused by CPT-1. The acyl-CoA is then available for the first reaction of β-oxidation.

currency of lipid metabolism. Acetyl-CoA is used for energy production in the mitochondria by the process known as the tricarboxylic acid cycle (TCA cycle), or the Krebs cycle. The TCA cycle takes acetyl-CoA and eventually turns it into the major energy currency of cells, namely adenosine triphosphate (ATP). Acetyl-CoA is the substrate for synthesis of ketone bodies. The start-

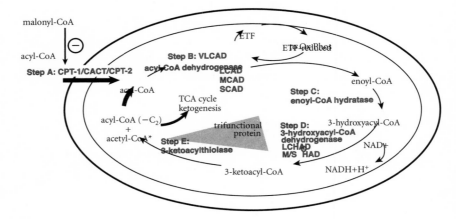

Figure 9.3. Overview of the cycle of mitochondrial β-oxidation of fatty acids. This process begins with transfer of acyl-CoA, a fatty acid substrate, from outside the mitochondrial membranes into the inner matrix of the mitochondrion. This occurs through the action of carnitine palmitoyltransferase-1 (CPT-1), carnitine-acylcarnitine translocase (CACT), and carnitine palmitoyltransferase-2 (CPT-2) (Step A, see also Figure 9.2). The acyl-CoA is first acted on by an acyl-CoA dehydrogenase (Step B). Four possible enzymes—which one depends on the chain length of the acyl-CoA—catalyze this single step. These enzymes include very long-chain acyl-CoA dehydrogenase (VLCAD), long-chain acyl-CoA dehydrogenase (LCAD), medium-chain acyl-CoA dehydrogenase (MCAD), and short-chain acyl-CoA dehydrogenase (SCAD). Next, in Step C, formation of 3-hydroxyacyl-CoA is catalyzed by enoyl-CoA hydratase; this product is then acted on by a 3-hydroxyacyl-CoA dehydrogenase (Step D). There are at least two 3-hydroxyacyl-CoA dehydrogenase enzymes, a long-chain structure (LCHAD) and a medium- or short-chain structure (M/SCHAD). A 3-ketoacyl-CoA is formed and the last step is accomplished by a 3-ketoacyl-CoA thiolase (Step E) that cleaves off an acetyl-CoA and an acyl-CoA two carbon units shorter. The acyl-CoA returns to the acyl-CoA dehydrogenase step for another round in this pathway. As it gets shorter, the enzyme with shorter chain-length specificity will take action for completing these steps. The final end product is acetyl-CoA, which is used for energy production and for ketogenesis. ETF, electron transport flavoprotein; Ox Phos, oxidative phosphorylation; NAD, NADH, nicotinamide adenine dinucleotide (+ H = reduced form); TCA, tricarboxylic acid cycle, also known as the Krebs cycle. The trifunctional protein is a complex of three enzymes used in the β-oxidation cycle—hydratase, LCHAD, and thiolase.

ing point of ketone body synthesis is the production of acetyl-CoA from fatty acid oxidation. The ketoacidosis that occurs in people with insulin-dependent (type 1) diabetes mellitus (Chapter 6) occurs because fatty acid β-oxidation has gone out of control and overproduced acetyl-CoA, resulting in overproduction of ketone bodies. Restrained ketone body synthesis (ketosis) in response to fasting or starvation is a normal process, but when it gets out of control and becomes excessive, as in diabetes, it can be a fatal.

The Spiral of Fatty Acid β-Oxidation

I am going to give a fair amount of detail on this process because the details will be important for later discussion of the serious diseases that occur as a result of deficiencies in these steps. Fatty acid β-oxidation is often described as a spiral process (Figure 9.4). A very long chain acyl-CoA enters the spiral at the top and, through a series of enzymatic steps, becomes shorter; the acyl-CoA then starts the cycle over, as an acyl-CoA that is two carbons shorter and is lower on the path of the spiral. The cycle continues down the spiral, each time with enzymes with shorter chain-length specificity. That is, this is not a simple cycle (Figure 9.3) that remains constant as it repeats, but rather a spiral of cy-

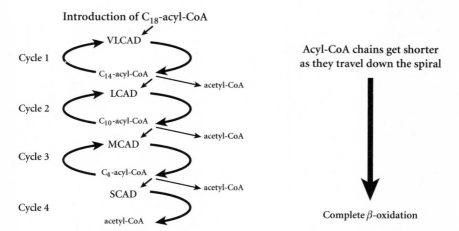

Figure 9.4. The spiral of mitochondrial β-oxidation of fatty acids. The enzymatic steps depicted in Figure 9.3 occur throughout each cycle at each level of the spiral shown here. After each cycle the fatty acid substrate is two carbons shorter than it was at the beginning. Finally, acetyl-CoA (with two carbons) is the end product.

cles that are slightly different in nature with each repetition. As the acyl-CoAs continue down this spiral, they get shorter as more and more usable energy is extracted in the process. In the end, the final product is acetyl-CoA and other energy intermediates: the reduced electron transport flavoprotein (ETF) and nicotinamide adenine dinucleotide reduced (NADH+H$^+$), shown in Figure 9.3. You might think of this process as a roller-coaster ride that drops from the highest point (the long-chain acyl-CoA) through a series of spiral turns (each one resulting in a smaller chain) before coming to rest at the bottom (Figure 9.4). A great deal of energy is extracted from this process of "falling" down this spiral.

The action begins at the acyl-CoA dehydrogenation step (Figure 9.3, Step B). For discussion here, let's assume the fatty acid is a C_{18}, the saturated fatty acid known as stearic acid or stearate. As soon as the acyl-CoA is regenerated from the imported acylcarnitine, it goes to the first dehydrogenase, called very long chain acyl-CoA dehydrogenase (VLCAD). Through the action of this enzyme, a double bond is introduced in the fatty acid molecule and the first energy equivalent is produced. As the double bond is produced, an electron is extracted from the chemical reaction and passed to another protein, the electron transport flavoprotein (ETF). This ETF is now "reduced" by the addition of the electron, and it can go on to another process, oxidative phosphorylation (Ox Phos). Oxidative phosphorylation is a key process for making ATP from the reduced, energy-containing ETF molecules (or, at later steps, from NADH). Another point about this step is that both the acyl-CoA dehydrogenase and the ETF contain a "flavin" component that is derived from the B-vitamin riboflavin. Let's get back to the spiral. The acyl-CoA at this point has been dehydrogenated and a double bond now exists at the second and third carbon position; at the same time, it has generated potential energy by reducing ETF.

After the action of VLCAD, the acyl-CoA with a double bond, now called an enoyl-CoA, is acted upon by the next enzyme in the step, enoyl-CoA hydratase (Figure 9.3, Step C), in which a water molecule is introduced to make a 3-hydroxy-acyl-CoA. This changes the double bond back to a single bond but also puts an OH or "hydroxy" group on the very end of the molecule. The long-chain 3-hydroxy-acyl-CoA is then acted upon by the next enzyme, long-chain 3-hydroxy-acyl-CoA dehydrogenase (LCHAD, see Figure 9.3, Step D). The next molecule produced is a 3-keto-acyl-CoA; the single bond between the OH group has now been made into a double bond, a structure that is reflected in the prefix *keto*.

The final step for this first cycle (Figure 9.4, Cycle 1) of the spiral of fatty acid oxidation is the 3-ketothiolase step (Figure 9.3, Step E), where the 3-keto-acyl-CoA is split into an acetyl-CoA and an acyl-CoA (C_{16}) two carbons shorter than the starting C_{18}-fatty acid, stearic acid. Because the three enzymes—hydratase, LCHAD, and thiolase—are found together as a complex, they have been called trifunctional protein. The acetyl-CoA can now go on to further energy production via the TCA cycle or be made into ketone bodies.

At this point, the acyl-CoA (C_{16}) will continue for an additional round at Cycle 1 before going further down the spiral. As the acyl-CoA gets shorter going from C_{16} to C_{14}, in the first cycle, a similar but distinct enzyme known as long-chain acyl-CoA dehydrogenase (LCAD, see Figure 9.4, Cycle 2) will dehydrogenate the bulk of the acyl-CoA (C_{14}) in Cycle 2 further down the spiral. It is unknown whether there are chain-length-specific enoyl-CoA hydratases, but there appears to be a medium/short-chain 3-hydroxy-acyl-CoA dehydrogenase (M/SCHAD) in addition to the already mentioned LCHAD. M/SCHAD will work on the shorter 3-hydroxy-acyl-CoAs when they are generated further down the spiral. As far as biochemists know, there is only one thiolase with no chain-length specificity. So on the process goes; after the acyl-CoA (C_{14}) has completed its turn down the spiral it will be acyl-CoA (C_{12}) (Figure 9.4). As it approaches C_{10} size, it will be dehydrogenated in the first step of Cycle 3, by medium-chain acyl-CoA-dehydrogenase (MCAD) along with other medium-range enzymes. Finally, as it approaches C_4-acyl-CoA size, at the bottom of the spiral, it will be dehydrogenated in the first step of Cycle 4 (Figure 9.4) by short-chain acyl-CoA dehydrogenase (SCAD) and the shorter-range enzymes.

Different genes encode each of these enzymes. I have mentioned chain-length specificity because in some genetic diseases (Chapter 10) the enzyme with short-chain specificity may be deficient due to a genetic mutation, whereas the enzyme with the same action but with long-chain specificity is not deficient. Because of these differences in the steps in mitochondrial β-oxidation, dietary fat intake of the relatively longer-chain fatty acids (C_{16-18}) will have a different influence on disease processes than will intake of shorter-chain fatty acids. The shorter acyl-CoAs (C_4) are usually generated within the mitochondria and not directly influenced by dietary fat.

The original C_{18}-acyl-CoA went down the spiral of steps—involving very long chain, long-chain, medium-chain, and short-chain enzymes—until it had been converted into nine acetyl-CoA molecules. These acetyl-CoAs will go on to be further used within the mitochondria for energy production by the TCA cycle or to be made into ketone bodies for energy export and glucose conservation.

This ends our overview of the metabolism of fatty acids and the cycles of buildup, breakdown, and burning of the fatty acids that make up triglycerides. I went into some detail about these processes because the key to understanding and doing something effective about diseases of excess fat is to understand where the fat comes from and where it goes. The next chapter builds on the present topic of fatty acid oxidation by exploring the diseases that result when one of the required enzymes is deficient as a result of a mutation. We then move on to the ways geneticists study genes that influence fat metabolism and the development of diseases of excess fat.

CHAPTER 10

Single-Gene Disorders of Lipid Metabolism

This chapter provides an overview of how changes in a single gene influence lipid metabolism and the body fat phenotype, in both normal and disease states. It explores the genetically simple, single-gene disorders that often have the most drastic effects on body size and health. These diseases are known as inborn errors of metabolism, many of which are severe in nature and very challenging to treat. This information will provide the groundwork for understanding the genetically complex, multifactorial diseases discussed in the next chapter.

Much of what we have learned about gene-metabolism relationships has come from studying inherited diseases of lipid metabolism. These are usually rare disorders that have profound abnormalities. Since these abnormalities are so distinct, they are relatively straightforward to decipher. As described next, an example is the discovery of the LDL receptor by Goldstein and Brown while studying patients with familial hypercholesterolemia (Goldstein, Hobbs, and Brown 2001). In its most severe form, FH causes abnormally elevated blood cholesterol and even heart attacks in teenagers and younger children. Oftentimes in the families of these children there is a history of having very high cholesterol in the blood and heart attacks among family members in their forties and fifties, a sign that something is very wrong with their cholesterol metabolism.

I will take a similar approach as my mode of explanation of the genetic determinants of normal fat metabolism. That is, I will explain the genetically simple disorders first—what have been called "experiments of Nature"—and then lead into a discussion of the multifactorial, multigene disorders that are most common.

Cholesterol Metabolism

There are some very severe diseases involving cholesterol metabolism in which lowering dietary cholesterol has virtually no effect. These are inherited diseases of cholesterol metabolism in which some key function in clearing cholesterol from the bloodstream or properly transporting it around the body in lipoproteins has been severely disrupted because of a genetic change. Studies of these relatively rare diseases have been helpful in genetically dissecting the key elements of cholesterol metabolism. The much more common, multifactorial diseases of cholesterol metabolism—referred to as garden-variety diseases of lipid metabolism back in Chapter 4—are more difficult to associate with a clear cause.

What I want to cover here are the relatively rare, but very serious, diseases of cholesterol metabolism that are genetically determined. Diet, exercise, and drugs may be helpful in the control of these extreme diseases, but oftentimes environmental modifications fail to correct the problem because some fundamental deficiency or malfunction in a genetically determined factor has occurred. Increased risk for heart attacks at an unusually early age is a common feature of some of these diseases, but not the only one. A conspicuous clinical feature that occurs in many, but not all, persons with these diseases is the development of bumps filled with lipid (mostly cholesterol) on tendons or under the skin surface. Some forms that are rich in cholesterol esters are called cutaneous (skin) or tendonous xanthomas. Another type of xanthomas, rich in triglycerides, are known as eruptive xanthomas because they may break open.

Familial Hypercholesterolemia—a Prototypical Inherited Disease of Cholesterol Metabolism

The most well known and best-studied inherited disease of cholesterol metabolism is familial hypercholesterolemia (FH). One in 500 individuals is a genetic carrier of this disease. This disease was thoroughly described by the spectacular, Nobel Prize–winning research of Michael Brown and Joseph Goldstein and their colleagues in Dallas, along with many other scientists in other laboratories (Goldstein, Hobbs, and Brown 2001). This research is a

prototype for learning about normal biology from a disease state using a genetic approach. What these research investigators discovered was that FH was
the result of mutations that caused a deficiency of LDL receptors. Chapter 4
described how these receptors are essential for retrieving cholesterol from the
blood, especially LDL cholesterol. Patients who are heterozygous for LDL receptor deficiency—that is, have one normal gene and one mutated gene—
have approximately half the normal number of these receptors. These folk often have a family history of relatively early heart attacks as well as markedly elevated blood cholesterol concentrations (350–550 mg/dl). Individuals who are
homozygous for LDL receptor deficiency—have two defective genes—have
extremely high blood cholesterol concentrations (650–1,000 mg/dl). Such persons may have heart attacks as children and may not live to the age of 20.
Treatment in these most severe cases may include drastic measures, such as
liver and heart transplants. In addition to identifying the single genes that
cause FH, the research by Goldstein and Brown led to further understanding
of entirely new concepts of gene regulation of the steps of cholesterol biosynthesis (Brown and Goldstein 1997).

My intention here is not to give a full review of the inherited diseases of
cholesterol metabolism. A summary of the archetypical diseases, their primary deficiencies, and the resulting characteristics is given in Table 10.1. I will
focus this discussion on key concepts that were learned from these genetic
diseases—for more details, see Rader (1996), Gotto (1999), Mayes (2000),
Brunzell and Deeb (2001), Kane and Havel (2001), and Mahley and Rall
(2001).

If you refer to the apolipoprotein components and functions of the lipoproteins described in Table 4.1, you may in many cases predict what diseases
would result from a genetic defect in producing the lipoprotein. For example,
if LDL receptors are deficient, then LDL cholesterol concentration will be abnormally high, as is the case for FH. Likewise, if lipoprotein lipase is deficient,
then we would predict that blood triglyceride concentrations would be abnormally high since lipoprotein lipase is the enzyme needed for stripping the fatty
acids away from the triglycerides carried by the lipoproteins (chylomicrons
and VLDLs). When a failure in a gene function results in low levels of apoA-I,
an essential component of HDL, levels of HDL cholesterol, the good cholesterol, fall in turn. These examples are clear links between a molecular "lesion"
at the gene level and a disease process at the organism level. Many excellent
books and chapters have been written about the details of these diseases. My

main goal here is to provide a brief glimpse of these rare diseases of choles-terol metabolism caused by a primary gene mutation, for they have helped de-fine the components of the cholesterol metabolism pathway.

Diet modifications and drugs sometimes alleviate these diseases, but in in-dividuals who lack the normal instructions for making key pieces of the body's metabolic functions, these treatments are far from curative. These dis-eases will show up in families, and biochemical or molecular genetic testing can screen many of these deficiencies, once correctly diagnosed. Through such screening, genetic risks could be determined. The more common diseases of cholesterol have some genetic component, but the genetic diseases I will dis-cuss here have a one-to-one correspondence between a normal gene function (or lack thereof) and a metabolic disorder. The common diseases are likely the result of the inheritance of multiple disease-causing alleles at many loci en-coding for the myriad of steps in cholesterol metabolism. The combination of these complex genetic traits with a diet high in cholesterol and saturated fat will produce a garden-variety hypercholesterolemia but, unlike those de-scribed in Table 10.1, the mechanisms of the disease may not be clearly iden-tified.

Deficient Fatty Acid Oxidation and Sudden Death

Fatty acid oxidation is more than just the body burning fat to keep us trim. It is essential for life, especially during periods of fasting or starvation. The heart normally burns fatty acids at all times for a majority of its energy production. I now want to describe briefly the inherited diseases of mitochondrial fatty acid oxidation and their extreme effects, usually found in children, such as sudden death, cardiac disease, fatty liver (Figure 10.1), and fasting intolerance. For the most part, these life-threatening diseases can be prevented by avoid-ance of fasting.

Many people are familiar with sudden infant death syndrome (SIDS). SIDS remains a medical riddle for which many answers have been proposed and few yet proven. SIDS is not a single disease or condition but the name given to deaths with unknown causes in infants or young children under a year of age. A small portion of SIDS cases are associated with inborn or inherited de-ficiencies in fatty acid oxidation. These babies die suddenly because they are unable to withstand going without food or tolerating a "fast." Older children and adults "fast" when they don't eat for periods longer than the usual time between meals, about five or six hours, though usually fasting is defined as go-

Table 10.1. Some rare but highly informative inherited disorders of lipid metabolism

Disease name (primary defect)	Effects on blood lipids	Basic mechanism
Familial hypercholesterolemia (LDL receptor deficiency)	Children and adults show markedly elevated total and LDL cholesterol	With a reduction (~50% in heterozygotes) or total absence (homozygotes) of LDL receptors, LDL cholesterol uptake is deficient in tissues, including liver, required for disposal of cholesterol
Lipoprotein lipase (LPL) deficiency (lipoprotein lipase deficiency)	Children and adults have markedly elevated chylomicrons resulting in elevated triglycerides and cholesterol and decreased LDL and HDL particles	Deficient LPL results in decreased clearance of chylomicrons and VLDL particles because the triglyceride load is not lipolyzed properly
ApoC-II deficiency (apoC-II deficiency)	Children and adults have elevated chylomicrons and VLDLs, resulting in elevated triglycerides and cholesterol and decreased HDL particles	ApoC-II deficiency is similar to LPL deficiency since apoC-II is involved in activating LPL
Familial dysbeta-lipoproteinemia (apoE deficiency)	Children and adults may have increased triglycerides and cholesterol	Deficiency of apoE disrupts the normal catabolism of remnant lipoprotein particles that require apoE for uptake and disposal, such as those derived from chylomicron and VLDL particles
Hepatic lipase deficiency (hepatic lipase (HL) deficiency)	Children and adults may have elevated triglycerides, cholesterol, and HDL	HL deficiency leads to elevated VLDL remnants and triglyceride-rich HDL particles

Table 10.1 (continued)

Disease name (primary defect)	Effects on blood lipids	Basic mechanism
ApoA-I deficiency (apoA-I deficiency)	Normal to elevated triglycerides, normal total cholesterol, decreased HDL cholesterol at all ages	Deficient apoA-I results in deficient HDL particles with normal chylomicrons and VLDL
LCAT deficiency, fish-eye disease/corneal opacity (lecithin cholesterol acyltransferase (LCAT) deficiency)	Elevated cholesterol and triglycerides in adults, low HDL cholesterol at all ages	Normal HDL particles cannot be assembled and reverse transport of cholesterol is reduced
Abeta-lipoproteinemia (microsomal transfer protein (MTP) deficiency)	Abnormally low total cholesterol and triglycerides in children and adults	ApoB-containing lipoproteins (chylomicrons, VLDL, LDL) cannot be assembled so cells are unable to absorb fat-soluble vitamins
Hypobeta-lipoproteinemia (defective apoB)	Unusually low blood cholesterol and triglycerides and abnormal HDL particles in children and adults	Deficiency of apoB-containing lipoproteins affecting mostly VLDL and LDL particles, but with assembly of chylomicrons and adequate vitamin absorption in heterozygotes; homozygotes may have more severe disease resembling abeta-lipoproteinemia

Note: These are monogenic diseases that unless otherwise noted are mild to nonexistent in heterozygous individuals.

ing without food for a time period of at least overnight. Infants under six months, however, must feed or nurse on demand. For some infants that's every two or three hours. In order to maintain its energy supply during these fasting periods, the body switches from glucose to stored fat as a source of fuel (see Chapter 9). Fatty acid oxidation takes place in the intracellular mitochondria and peroxisomes via specific pathways.

As discussed in Chapter 9 (Figures 9.3 and 9.4), fatty acid oxidation pathways are composed of a series of chemical reactions mediated by enzymes that function to carry out each step along the way and ultimately generate a large amount of energy in the form of ATP. The heart uses fatty acid oxidation for energy a majority of the time, but during periods of fasting the liver and other organs that normally oxidize glucose will switch to this method of energy production as well. After a prolonged fast, when most of the glucose stored as glycogen has been depleted, hormone signals such as insulin (low) and glucagon (high) are both signaling that fat must be burned and that glucose not only must be conserved but also must be generated in the liver and kidney by gluconeogenesis. This is a process whereby amino acids generated from protein breakdown, which come predominantly from muscle, are converted into glucose by the liver and kidney. It is an energy-consuming process: as the liver burns fatty acids it uses the resulting energy to generate glucose via gluconeogenesis. This is an important process because unless blood glucose is maintained at a sufficient concentration a person may lose consciousness.

The other critical product of fat burning is the generation of ketone bodies.

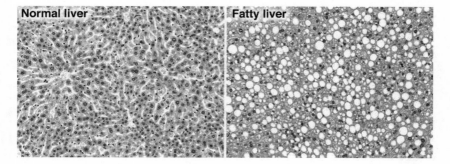

Figure 10.1. Microscopic sections of livers from a normal mouse *(left)* and a mouse with an inherited deficiency in fatty acid oxidation *(right)*. The fat deposits appear as open, empty vacuoles. Similarly high amounts of fat may be present in the livers of obese human subjects and those developing NASH. (Photograph courtesy of Trenton R. Schoeb.)

In acute episodes of insulin-dependent type 1 diabetes, the generation of excessive ketone bodies *(ketoacidosis)* is at life-threatening overabundance. In contrast, the inborn diseases of fatty acid oxidation, where fatty acids cannot be fully oxidized and turned into ketone bodies, result in a life-threatening deficiency of ketogenesis. Ketone bodies are an alternative fuel source for muscle and other organs, like the brain; the burning of ketones spares the glucose that is already in short supply. In babies with an inborn enzyme deficiency in the fatty acid oxidation pathway, the decreased ability to use fatty acids after a period without feeding results in a cellular energy deficiency and, eventually, in a dangerous buildup of fatty acids and toxic metabolites. Thus in the short term, they have a life-threateningly drastic decrease in blood glucose (hypoglycemia), and at the same time they have a deficient capacity to generate the ketone bodies that normally help compensate for hypoglycemia. The collection of clinical abnormalities—including hypoglycemia, elevated blood ammonia concentrations, and fatty deposits in the liver—is often called Reye-like disease because of the similarity to Reye syndrome. These acute disorders are only part of the major metabolic challenges facing these children.

Children with fatty acid oxidation (FAO) enzyme deficiencies may suffer from cardiac problems. This makes sense, as we know that the heart relies on FAO to meet its energy demands. FAO-deficient hearts, which somehow have adapted to functioning during a fed or unstressed state, are now challenged not only by an energy deficiency but also by the buildup of normal metabolites, acylcarnitines and acyl-CoAs, that may become toxic in excess. Some of these effects can be readily seen through the microscope as droplets of triglyceride in the hearts of mice that also have inborn deficiencies in fatty acid oxidation (Kurtz et al. 1998; Cox et al. 2001). Acylcarnitines are natural compounds but are usually present in very low concentrations. It has been postulated that human patients with deficiencies in fatty acid oxidation generate excessive concentrations of acylcarnitines in the heart, and these compounds are a suspected cause of cardiac arrhythmia.

Fasting, which requires intact mitochondrial fatty acid oxidation for energy production while sparing glucose, is the primary challenge to children with inborn errors of mitochondrial fatty acid oxidation. The full-spectrum acute disease that occurs is characterized by metabolic acidosis and elevated fatty acids in the blood. Children with enzyme deficiencies that impair oxidation of longer-chain fatty acids, such as very long chain acyl-CoA dehydrogenase, may suffer heart disease: acute cardiac arrhythmia and possible sudden death or more chronic changes, such as development of an enlarged heart *(cardiac hy-*

pertrophy). These problems result from energy imbalances within the heart muscle rather than from a restricted blood flow, the culprit commonly associated with coronary artery disease and heart attacks.

Missing Steps of Mitochondrial Fatty Acid Oxidation

Different enzyme deficiencies are included in this group of diseases because any of the different steps of mitochondrial fatty acid oxidation may be disrupted (Wood 1999; Roe and Ding 2001). Long-chain fatty acid substrates (C_{16-20}) for fatty acid oxidation are derived from the diet, while the short-chain fatty acid substrates (C_{4-14}) are predominantly generated within the mitochondria. In general, when steps involving the long-chain fatty acids are deficient, the overall disease is more severe; long-chain fatty acid oxidation deficiencies tend to cause long-term or chronic heart disease, in addition to the acute diseases described earlier. In contrast, patients with short-chain fatty acid oxydation deficiencies have the advantage of burning their long-chain fatty acids down through the top part of the fatty acid oxidation spiral (Figure 9.4). If, however, there is a long-chain fatty acid oxydation defect and most incoming fatty acids are long-chain, then oxidation is stopped at the very beginning of the spiral. Since there are only small amounts of short-chain fatty acids available in the conventional diet or stored in adipose tissue, there are essentially no substrates available to enter lower in the spiral and bypass the block.

The specific enzyme deficiencies known in human patients are shown in Table 10.2. If you compare this table with Figure 9.3, you can see the connections between the deficient steps and where in the pathway the fatty acid oxidation stops. The initial deficiencies discovered in this pathway were mainly the acyl-CoA dehydrogenase deficiencies. Medium-chain acyl-CoA dehydrogenase (MCAD) deficiency is the most common one, especially in Caucasians of northern European descent (Roe and Ding 2001). A specific mutant allele occurs in this population at a rate of 1/60 to 1/100 individuals as genetic carriers. Many people have heard of phenylketonuria (PKU) because all states screen newborn babies for this inherited enzyme deficiency of amino acid metabolism at birth. MCAD deficiency is almost as common an inherited metabolic disease in Caucasians as PKU is in the general population. As patients were found to have some sort of fatty acid oxidation disease, enzyme deficiencies elsewhere in the pathway were discovered.

One of the mysteries of these diseases is that when the affected children grow into adolescence, they become more resistant to disease episodes. They

Table 10.2. Human enzyme deficiencies of mitochondrial β-oxidation of fatty acids

Enzyme deficiency	Common clinical characteristics	Common biochemical characteristics
Short-chain acyl-CoA dehydrogenase (SCAD)	Neonatal form, acute, potentially fatal disease; milder adult forms with wide range of possible phenotypes	Hypoketonemia / hypoglycemia; ethylmalonic aciduria
Medium-chain acyl-CoA dehydrogenase (MCAD)	Fasting intolerance; Reye-like syndrome; sudden death	Hypoketonemia / hypoglycemia; hyperammonemia
Long-chain acyl-CoA dehydrogenase (LCAD)	None known; previously mistaken for VLCAD deficiency	Unknown
Very long-chain acyl-CoA dehydrogenase (VLCAD)	Hypertrophic cardiomyopathy; Reye-like syndrome; sudden death	Hypoketonemia / hypoglycemia
Long-chain hydroxyacyl-CoA dehydrogenase (LCHAD) / Trifunctional protein	Severe acute liver disease; hypertrophic cardiomyopathy, retinopathy; fatty liver pregnancy / HELLP syndrome (hypertension, elevated liver enzymes, low platelets)	Hypoketonemia / hypoglycemia; 3-hydroxydicarboxylic aciduria
Short-chain hydroxyacyl-CoA dehydrogenase (SCHAD)	Myoglobinuria; encephalopathy; hypertrophic cardiomyopathy	Hypoketonemia / hypoglycemia

do not necessarily become totally resistant. As adults these individuals are able to transmit the genes for enzyme deficiency to their children, of course; genetic diagnosis and counseling then becomes very important.

Long-chain hydroxyacyl-CoA dehydrogenase (LCHAD) deficiency, further down the cycle, involves an additional and unusual complication not found in the other diseases. When a pregnant woman who is a genetic carrier of LCHAD deficiency carries a homozygous LCHAD-deficient fetus, she is likely to develop fatty liver of pregnancy and the so-called HELLP syndrome. HELLP syndrome is characterized by hypertension, elevated liver enzymes, and low platelets (Ibdah et al. 1999). This disease apparently develops because the fetus is producing toxic metabolites and the mother, who has a deficient capacity to metabolize them during pregnancy, cannot clear them. The fetus is excreting toxins into the mother's blood supply, across the placenta. Since this happens late in gestation, the only treatment is early delivery of the baby. Although this inherited enzyme deficiency is rare, this unusual complication occurs in about a third of pregnancies of this type.

Medical geneticists still have much to elucidate about the diseases of fatty acid oxidation, whose genesis and mechanisms remain cloudy. It is not unusual for pediatricians to find children with disease signs identical to those as I have described above, yet physicians and scientists have thus far failed to pinpoint which step in the chain of events that has gone awry. Likewise, scientists have not found patients with a deficiency of each of the known enzymatic steps. A very curious example is that no one has found a human patient with LCAD deficiency, whereas my research team has developed a mouse model for this deficiency (Kurtz et al. 1998). Scientists suspect either that LCAD deficiency is harmless in humans, is lethal to the gestating fetus, or is simply undiagnosed because it lacks the expected characteristics of a fatty acid oxidation disorder.

Enzyme Deficiency Diseases in a Family

A common problem is that parents are often unaware that their child has an inborn error of fatty acid oxidation until the child has the first acute disease episode from fasting. Another is that common childhood diseases such as a respiratory or gastrointestinal upset—basically, anything that induces the child to vomit or to not eat—will set off an acute disease episode without warning. Disease events due to an inherited enzyme deficiency are often an entire surprise to everyone, including the pediatrician. Fortunately, the overall chances of an inherited disease occurring are very low, since the inheritance of two uncommon deficiency alleles is extremely rare, but unlucky combinations do occur. Of course, neither parent was likely ever sick from having a single copy of the deficiency allele. Another tragedy of these inherited deficiencies is that only half of the affected babies survive if they have an acute disease episode.

Mouse models have also revealed a unique feature of these inherited enzyme deficiencies, and that is cold intolerance (Guerra et al. 1998). Mice rely on fatty acid oxidation in brown adipose tissue to maintain body temperature. Human babies likewise have significant amounts of brown adipose tissue, but whether cold intolerance is involved in sudden infant death remains to be defined. The best hope is that the disease is correctly diagnosed in the emergency room. Unfortunately, these rare diseases may look like some other, more common disease or severe illness, such as an infection. Often, children with an inborn error in fatty acid oxidation are misdiagnosed, and their severe energy deficiency and toxicity are not treated. A normal baby with severely low blood glucose concentrations will have a robust ketone body response, but these

---

The Case of the Unidentified Disorder of Fat Oxidation

The Moore family had three sons. Jason died at age three years, and his brother Jonathan died at age four years. Both had an undefined disorder of fatty acid oxidation. Both boys had the same disease characteristics: muscle wasting, fatty change in the liver, heart, and kidneys, and, eventually, cardiac arrhythmia and arrest. The third boy never showed any signs of the disease. (The family's story is told in Butgereit 1992). When the Moore sons were sick, diagnostic capabilities were not as advanced as they are today. Although tissue samples were sent to laboratories around the world for a specific biochemical diagnosis, none was determined. One of the Moore family's remaining concerns was the possibility of the same deficiency in the surviving brother. He most likely was not homozygous for the same disorder because he had not shown any signs of the early stages of his brothers' disease. He could be a genetic carrier for the deficiency, though. In any case like this, it means a great deal to the family to have a diagnosis and be able to give a name to the disorder that affected their loved ones. I later met Mr. Moore, and he remained optimistic that someday they would learn what disease took his sons.

children do not. The most important considerations for combatting these inherited diseases are correct diagnosis, prevention of fasting, and genetic screening and counseling of the other family members. Siblings have a high likelihood of being homozygous (1 in 4) or heterozygous (1 in 2) for one of these enzyme deficiencies if both parents are genetic carriers.

This discussion has centered on the extreme conditions of deficient fatty acid oxidation and the potential dire end results. Fortunately, if children with inborn deficiencies can be diagnosed early on, their health can be maintained by avoidance of fasting. It is interesting to see the obsessive-compulsive behaviors parents of these children will display as far as maintaining adequate caloric intake. There are extremes at both ends of the scale. Some parents are cavalier—they do not seem at all vigilant about feeding their children—and oftentimes they get away with it. Other parents never, no matter what, let their baby go for more than three or so hours, around the clock, without a feeding. As might be expected, some of those babies become obese, which means they may be at increased disease risk if they ever do fast because of the high dose of fatty acids that could be released, via lipolysis, from the excess fat. This may be a significant challenge to their compromised ability to burn the fatty acids released.

In many states newborn screening protocols include testing for inherited disorders of fatty acid oxidation, so there is a growing chance these children will be found before they have a life-threatening disease episode. Not only is it important to try to counter the deficiency, but if these children are sick from some other cause, they must not become energy depleted. That is, if they acquire an infectious disease and do not eat or have vomiting, they are at high risk of an acute disease episode. I have included this group of diseases as an example of the extreme conditions of genetic deficiency of fatty acid metabolism. This pathway of fatty acid oxidation is important in the overall balance of lipid metabolism.

The focus in this chapter has been on the single-gene disorders of cholesterol and fatty acid metabolism. As described, these are relatively clear-cut genetic disorders, although often difficult to treat. More commonly, metabolic diseases with abnormal lipid metabolism have multiple, yet subtle, genetic causes, and diet and activity level have significant roles in the overall disease character. The next chapter takes up the subject of complex or polygenic diseases and their effects on lipid metabolism.

CHAPTER 11

Multifactorial Genetic Diseases of Lipid Metabolism

The single-gene disorders discussed in Chapter 10 illustrate the genetic basis of metabolic pathology. Much more common, however, are disorders with multiple causes. Multifactorial diseases may involve not only more than one gene but also nongenetic factors, such as the environment and behavioral patterns. Geneticists are trying to put together the pieces of this complex puzzle and develop possible strategies for physicians in the future to use a patient's genetic profile in determining risk assessment, diagnosis, and treatment of these complex diseases. The goal is to base preventive care or treatment on genotype—in other words, to counter the effects of genetic differences with prescribed diet, activity level, drugs, or other measures.

Mendelian Inheritance

In this chapter, I describe for you a set of individuals with a hypothetical set of genotypes and a variety of lipid characteristics. A genotype is simply the set of genes, estimated at around 30–40,000 genes, inherited by an individual from each parent. Each individual has two copies (alleles) of every gene. If an allele is shared by a large majority of the population (>99%), it is described as a "wild-type" or "normal" allele. Mutations occasionally change the molecular structure of an allele and therefore alter its function. Mutant alleles are passed down through generations, as normal alleles are, and eventually may occur in some proportion of the population. A single-gene disorder is caused by the inheritance of at least one allele that is not "normal"—in the case of familial hypercholesterolemia (FH), one or both alleles of the LDL-receptor gene is a mutant. To get the most severe effects of the disease, a person must inherit a mutant (or "variant") allele from both mother and father; such a person is *homozygous* for the LDL-receptor mutation. A person who inherits one mutant allele and one normal allele is *heterozygous* for this mutant allele and will also have a dangerously elevated blood cholesterol concentration, but it will not be as severe as a homozygous patient. Since the disease occurs when a person inherits only one mutant allele, FH is considered a *dominant* disease. (If a normal allele could carry out the gene's function even if the other allele was a mutant, the mutation is described as *recessive*.)

FH is a good illustration of what has been called the "gene dosage effect." Having one mutant LDL-receptor allele is bad, but having two is worse. It is an "all or none" scenario: it hardly matters what other genes were inherited, since the LDL-receptor deficiency is not compensated for by other genes or other remedies. That is, there are no other genes that can provide the instructions for synthesizing the needed LDL receptors, and even a low-cholesterol diet will not overcome the strong effect that inheriting mutant LDL-receptor genes has on the patient.

The disease traits discussed in the previous chapter follow the simple inheritance patterns described in the nineteenth century by Gregor Mendel. Basically, this means that the disease traits follow a pattern of dominant or recessive inheritance while other genes or environmental factors have minor effects in modifying the disease phenotype (the physical characteristics of an individual). The Mendelian traits that were emphasized in the last chapter are also known as monogenic or single-gene traits.

In contrast to monogenic disease traits, multifactorial disease traits—often called polygenic, multigenic, or complex diseases—occur when variant alleles of multiple genes are not so drastically different from wild-type alleles but their differences do disturb the body's functions. The degree of disease depends on the collective function or dysfunction of other genes inherited. That is, many monogenic traits are caused by a complete deficiency of function in a particular gene product, like the absence of LDL receptors caused by FH. In contrast, complex traits, such as development of high blood lipids or diabetes, occur as a result of genetic differences in alleles within "quantitative trait loci (genes)." Variant alleles within quantitative trait loci may encode for an enzyme that has 60% of normal function rather than a complete absence of function. These may be relatively subtle changes, but they add up! That is, in order for a person to develop the common dyslipidemias, such as hypercholesterolemia, combinations of subtle gene changes add up to produce these disease traits. The gene products affected by the dysfunctional alleles may include a wide array of proteins with many different types of functions. The gene products that determine a person's lipid phenotype may include enzymes (e.g., HMG-CoA reductase), receptors (LDL receptor), transcription factors (PPAR-α), or hormones (leptin). Quite likely, however, genes that are yet to be discovered may encode for proteins with functions we never knew about before. Therefore, the genetic pathogenesis of multifactorial diseases will likely involve not only the coding sequences of genes and their immediate products, but also downstream effects on gene regulation. Other genes can encode for proteins that regulate other genes (on/off switches) or their level of expression (controlling the "volume"). If, in addition to these genetic intricacies, the particular diet and exercise habits of a person are considered, we then have a very complex situation to sort out.

You will also hear the term *penetrance* with regard to genetic influences on phenotype. Not all individuals with a given genotype always show the same phenotype. Geneticists who study entire populations may find that some people show a given trait quite robustly while others show it mildly or not at all, even though all the individuals inherited the same allele for the gene of interest. Each individual is counted either plus or minus for the trait. The individuals showing varying degrees of the disease phenotype are showing variable *expressivity* with regard to inheriting the gene (allele) of interest. Therefore, penetrance refers to how many individuals in a population that shares a particular allele of a gene show the disease trait (mild to severe), while expressivity refers to whether an individual with a particular allele expresses a mild or severe form of the disease.

Gene interactions may be favorable, neutral, or unfavorable. Table 11.1 presents the gene combinations for six patients, along with their "net lipid phenotype." Of course, the patient's age, sex, ancestry, diet, and exercise habits will all affect the net outcome. There is a certain "genetic tipping point" where, given the person's genotype plus their environment and behavior, disease will occur. Let's assume exercise and diet are similar for these patients—all we know is that blood lipid abnormalities seem to run in their families. How do we make sense of the complexity of the genetics involved? It is like taking a trip to London. You know that when you get there you will see the Tower of London, Parliament, Westminster Abbey, and the rest, but you are sitting at the moment in Dodge City, Kansas. You will have to travel by car to Wichita, Kansas, board an airplane and fly to New York, where you board another plane to fly to London. We know here what types of genes we are looking for in the end—namely, those affecting lipid metabolism—but we are going to have to plan a strategy to make our way through multiple points to end up with the genetic information we are pursuing.

For the patients in Table 11.1, I have created hypothetical genetic profiles. Shirley, for example, happens to be homozygous wild-type for "Normal Lipids Gene A" but heterozygous for the mutant form of Gene B. There may be no net effect, because Gene A compensates for Gene B's half-dose of dysfunction. For Richard, whose Gene A and Gene B are both heterozygous, there may be trouble. A high proportion of individuals with this theoretical genotype will develop a moderate elevation in blood cholesterol concentrations. Carol is in the more common situation. She has heterozygosity at Genes A and B, like Richard, but she has several other mutant genes that affect fat metabolism. Her cholesterol is slightly higher than Richard's. It gets even more complicated because Carol is a premenopausal woman and Richard is a man of the same age, illustrating the significant effects of sex and age. So even with her other gene changes, the rise in cholesterol was only a little more in Carol, perhaps because Richard did not have the protective advantage of estrogen. The other possibility is that if these patients' blood cholesterol concentrations were measured on another day, they might even be equal. Normal daily fluctuations in blood lipid concentrations could cause such a result. Mark is the son of Richard. He has somewhat better cholesterol values because, although he inherited the same mutant alleles for Genes A and B, he inherited a double dose of "Lipid-Lowering Gene D," unlike his father (Richard).

These examples show how hard it is to figure out the causes and effects of various diseases. Patients with FH (like Albert in our example), however, can do very little to change their blood cholesterol concentrations because this single gene defect is so powerful. That is, this mutation has high penetrance: Virtually everyone in the population who has the mutant allele has the disease. Since a person needs only one of the two genes for LDL-receptor synthesis to be mutated to develop the disease, this is a dominant trait. The other genes (Genes A–G) in Table 11.1 have very subtle and possibly additive effects on the overall phenotype of blood cholesterol concentrations.

The more common but less well defined types of hyperlipidemia remain difficult to sort out genetically. Also, there are genotypes that probably promote for elevated blood triglyceride and free fatty acid concentrations by affecting fatty acid metabolism directly. These effects, in turn, promote for insulin resistance and eventually diabetes as well. There is a genetic "domino

Table 11.1. Possible gene interactions resulting in the polygenic trait hypercholesterolemia

Patient/Age	Wild-type profile: Robert, age 35	F H patient: Albert, age 35	Patient 1: Shirley, age 25	Patient 2: Richard, age 38	Patient 3: Carol, age 38	Patient 4: Mark, age 16
Phenotype	Normal cholesterol: 150 mg/dl	High cholesterol: 285 mg/dl	Normal cholesterol: 150 mg/dl	Elevated cholesterol: 235mg/dl	Elevated cholesterol: 245mg/dl	Elevated cholesterol: 220mg/dl
Genes			Genotype			
LDL-receptor	+/+	+/−	+/+	+/+	+/+	+/+
Normal Lipids Gene A	+/+	+/+	+/+	+/−	+/−	+/−
Normal Lipids Gene B	+/+	+/+	+/−	+/−	+/−	+/−
Normal Lipids Gene C	+/+	+/+	+/+	+/+	+/+	+/+
Low Lipids Gene D	+/+	+/+	+/+	+/−	+/−	+/+
Normal Lipids Gene E	+/+	+/+	+/+	+/+	+/+	+/+
Low Lipids Gene F	+/+	+/+	+/+	+/+	−/−	+/+
Normal Lipids Gene G	+/+	+/+	+/+	+/+	+/+	+/+

Note: A plus (+) means that the allele is wild-type and functioning 100% to achieve the effect naming the gene. A minus (−) means the allele is a mutant or variant. If there is a + allele at Gene A, then it is functioning to contribute to normal blood lipid concentrations; if there is a + allele at Gene D, then it is functioning actively to lower effect." Clearly, there is a heritable component to type 2 diabetes. Studies with monozygotic twins have shown that 60–70% of identical twins develop diabetes if one twin has the disease, whereas dizygotic twins (not identical) have around a 10–20% co-occurrence of diabetes (Kahn and Porte 2001). The heritability of diabetes is highest in the Pima Indians of Arizona, where around 80% of offspring from parents who were both diabetic also develop the disease. Despite strong evidence of a genetic component, even in the Pimas, the clear-cut genes and the particular alleles involved that promote for diabetes have been extremely elusive.

So on one hand are the Mendelian disease traits like FH, cystic fibrosis, or sickle-cell anemia, and many others, where a clear and predictable pattern of disease results when mutant alleles are inherited. On the other hand, and in much higher frequency, are disease traits that are certainly inherited but result from a combination of factors. For these diseases it doesn't matter if the individual, like Richard, is homozygous or heterozygous for a single, particular "Normal Lipids Gene A." The answer might be that inheritance of a mutant Gene A must be combined with homozygous inheritance of "Normal Lipids Gene B," at least a heterozygous dose of "Normal Lipids Gene C," and, finally, the lipid-lowering allele for "Low Lipids Gene D." In addition to his genotype, other factors contribute to Richard's elevated cholesterol level. He eats around 50 grams of saturated fat along with over 200 grams of simple carbohydrates per day, and his only exercise is walking from the car to the office and back on any given day. With this combination of complex genotype, sedentary behavior, diet, Richard has fasting blood metabolite values as shown in Table 11.2. He is a typical dyslipidemic patient who is insulin resistant and diabetic. He also has high blood pressure (hypertension). He is the prototypical metabolic syndrome patient (Chapter 5).

Table 11.2. Fasting blood metabolite concentrations of Patient 2, Richard

Blood measurements	Concentration (mg/dl)	Desirable values
Total cholesterol	⇑ 358	< 200
VLDL cholesterol	⇑ 183	< 20
LDL cholesterol	⇑ 147	< 130
HDL cholesterol	⇓ 28	> 40
Triglycerides	⇑ 426	< 150
Glucose	⇑ 142	< 100
Blood pressure (mm of Hg)	⇑ 145/98	< 130/80

Richard also fits the combined hypercholesterolemia and hypertriglycer-idemia category described in Chapter 4. That is, he has high blood cholesterol and triglyceride concentrations, contained within high concentrations of LDL and VLDL particles.

A "reductionist" approach mandates that scientists decipher each component that makes up the metabolic character of this individual by breaking down each one into its simplest parts. This might be considered the "test tube" or "in vitro" approach to science. As one example, scientists might study in isolation the gene sequence of Normal Lipids Gene A. The context beyond the test tube, however, is critical. Thus, an "integrative" approach would take into account the isolated individual components (e.g., sequence of Normal Lipids Gene A) but also the context of the whole body and the environment. Biomedical science requires both approaches: a "reductionist" program to discover the functions of the individual components, followed by an "integrative" attempt to weave the component parts into a coherent explanation of lipid disorders. This strategy promises our best chance of preventing, treating, or even curing the disease.

Pursuing Genetic Complexity

Complex diseases like hypercholesterolemia result from the inheritance of many different genes with either normal function or dysfunction in different dosages ($+/-$ or $-/-$). Such diseases are further complicated by environmental influences, such as diet and activity level. One approach to understanding this genetic complexity is "gene mapping" using single nucleotide polymorphisms, or SNPs (pronounced "snips"). Variant alleles of genes that influence lipid metabolism (or any phenotype, for that matter) can be tagged by identifying SNPs linked with the genes of interest. SNPs are used to study the combinations of genes that contribute to the development of disease. SNPs are also being used to track down genes that seem to predict whether a particular drug may work well in some patients and be toxic in others. As shown for the hypothetical patients in Table 11.1, what if we could "detect and distinguish" each gene named in the left column and decipher a genotype pattern in real patients? Geneticists do not have to know what the genes do or how they do it, but they would know that if someone inherits this or that combination of particular alleles, that person would likely end up with modifications in their blood lipid values. Furthermore, what if geneticists could determine the differences among these alleles with a particular marker or "tag" of each? The SNPs serve first as a tag indicating a specific location within the genome. A SNP may explain a particular gene dysfunction, but most often it does not. The "SNP tagging" approach works because geneticists do not have to know anything about the genes to start searching for disease gene alleles. They often do not even know which chromosome the locus is on, what protein is encoded, let alone the sequence abnormalities that change the gene's function and result in disease.

So let's say we could analyze for the Normal Lipids Gene A in all the patients in Table 11.1. Each patient has two alleles of Gene A. In our example, patients have either a wild-type (normal) allele of Gene A, designated by a ($+$), or they have a mutant or variant allele, indicating deficiency, designated by a ($-$). Now, if geneticists could find a "tag" that would clearly distinguish the ($+$) allele of Gene A from the ($-$) allele of Gene A, they could follow these genes through families and study their genotype-phenotype (lipid disease characteristics) relationships. That's where SNPs come in.

SNPs are sequences of nucleotides in DNA molecules that in some individuals are different from the sequences in the large majority of the population. They provide an identifiable "tag" or "landmark" in the genome. A SNP might be directly involved in causing gene dysfunction, but the most common scenario is that it is a harmless difference in sequence that merely marks a gene that should be studied further. That is, the SNP may not have anything to do with the functional difference between a variant gene and the wild-type gene. It most likely is only a variation that is useful as a tag or marker for this different allele. For example, a gene with a sequence of CGGATAGCTTA could be the wild-type, while a sequence of CGGATGGCTTA could be the variant form. A single nucleotide variation would then be designated a SNP at that locus. If a variation occurs at this locus of a chromosome in more than 1% of the individuals in the population examined, it is considered a genetic polymorphism. When the sequence variation occurs in less than 1% of the loci examined, it is considered a rare variant. Geneticists determine the sequence from the wild-type allele and use it as the "standard." Then they compare it to the "polymorphism" or single nucleotide change in the variant alleles. SNPs are now widely used as markers for locations in the genome, and they can be used to follow genes in families. Furthermore, as discussed below, SNPs are used to detect disease-causing alleles out of the multitude of genetic loci on chromosomes.

Gene Sleuthing with SNPs

As noted above, SNPs may be used to tag genes or genomic segments of DNA from one person's genome and compare them to another's genome. Using this technology, geneticists follow specific alleles among family members or even among larger populations. Ideally, geneticists would identify all genes throughout the genome that influence development of abnormal lipid metabolism. Next, a multigene read-out could be produced on the basis of SNP ID tags for a given patient. With individualized genetic medicine, a physician in the future would know that the patient's problem is that she or he inherited two dysfunctional alleles of genes that should maintain normal lipids and no functional alleles that promote for lipid lowering (Table 11.1). In an ideal situation, they would know that this diet and that drug would be the best bet to lower the patient's lipids. That would happen in a perfect world. But how do we find the lipid metabolism genes to start with? And how do we use SNPs to identify the combination of genes that determine these complex phenotypes?

A major goal of the Human Genome Project (1990–2003) was to determine the sequence of the entire human genome. This project not only would provide a sequence of every gene but also would help us to understand the relationships of chromosomal locations. In addition, it provided a detailed gene map for hunting down disease-causing alleles in families. Despite the news media and even some scientists' impressions, the Human Genome Project is nothing more than an enormous tool to study human biology and disease. The genome project is not the end but a means to help in understanding diseases. We do not know how to cure every disease now that we have the genome sequence.

Human beings have 23 pairs of chromosomes, including the sex chromosomes X and Y. Each chromosome is a single, very long DNA molecule that is held together by various proteins. Coding segments, also known as exons, of genes make up very little of the total sequence of the genome. A lot of the rest has been called "junk" DNA, meaning that scientists simply do not yet know what it is for. It will probably turn out to be functional, so perhaps we should call it "enigma DNA." Nature is very frugal and usually does not allow any organism to carry around a lot of useless baggage. As far as gene hunting is concerned, finding a single gene in the mammoth amount of DNA contained in our genomes is like "looking for a needle in the haystack in the dark," as preeminent gene hunter Francis S. Collins (Director of the National Genome Research Institute) has said. SNPs have turned out to be a wonderful tool to search for genes that influence human traits.

The concept of a SNP occurring in different parts of a gene is demonstrated in Figures 11.1 and 11.2. The letters of the genome stand for adenine (A), cytosine (C), guanine (G), and thymine (T). Basic gene anatomy consists of exons, which are the coding sequences within a gene, and introns, the intervening sequences between the exons (Figure 11.2). Regulatory sequences, such as promoters, enhancers, and response elements, are most frequently found at the 5' end of the gene, which is usually depicted to the left of the first exon (Figure 11.2).

I will not describe how SNPs are determined in the laboratory because I want to concentrate, instead, on the way SNPs are used to find genes and eventually could be used for better diagnosis and treatment of lipid disorders. So let's start with the premise that we can determine a SNP profile representing 400 polymorphic loci throughout the genome. Beware that there are many more than that! These genomic regions will have known or unknown functions. By the way, *loci* is the plural form of *locus,* which simply means a "location" in the genome, either a gene location or simply a region of genomic sequence that has a SNP. From the human genome databases we could readily find 400 or many more loci defined by SNPs. There may be more than two choices of specific SNPs defining each allele. For example, Figure 11.2 shows four different alleles, each distinguished by a different SNP pattern. But let's

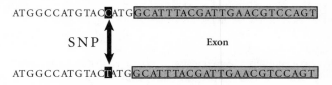

Single Nucleotide Polymorphisms - SNPs

SNP –1 "tags" Normal Lipids Gene A –functional allele

ATGGCCATGTAC**C**ATG GCATTTACGATTGAACGTCCAGT

SNP ↕   Exon

ATGGCCATGTAC**T**ATG GCATTTACGATTGAACGTCCAGT

SNP-2 "tags" Normal Lipids Gene A –dysfunctional allele

Figure 11.1. Illustrated here is the sequence for two alleles of the same gene, but with different "tags" identified by single nucleotide polymorphisms, or SNPs (highlighted). These two alleles could be distinguished among individuals in a study to establish a relationship between a particular allele of this gene and disease. The shaded areas represent coding sequences that are known as "exons."

assume there are only two possibilities, known here as SNP-allele 1 or SNP-allele 2.

Suppose we determine the SNP profile of 400 polymorphic loci in a large family that has a familial pattern of combined hypercholesterolemia and hypertriglyceridemia (i.e., high LDL cholesterol and high VLDL triglyceride concentrations). The 400 polymorphic loci were selected at random to do what geneticists call a genome scan. In actual studies many more SNPs are sampled. These loci will be distinguished by different SNP sequences, and these differences are located within or next to genes in regions that represent regulatory

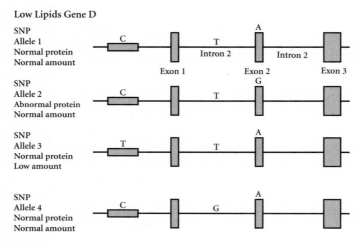

Figure 11.2. SNPs can occur anywhere in a segment of genomic DNA, including in a gene. Only the SNPs are shown as sequence. There are DNA sequences all along these segments, but unless indicated by the single-letter SNP, the sequences are identical in all four alleles shown. In other words, there are DNA letters (G, C, A, T) all along these segments (black lines) like those shown in Figure 11.1. Allele 1 is considered the normal or wild-type allele. Allele 2 has a polymorphism (A→G) in exon 2 (gray box) that turns out to be the mutation causing dysfunction. Allele 3 has a polymorphism (C→T) in the regulatory sequence (box at the left) of the gene that causes an abnormally low level of expression of an otherwise normal protein. That is, there are no changes in the coding sequence. Allele 4 has a polymorphism (T→G) within an intron (black line) that has no net functional effect on the gene. The function of this allele is identical with that of the wild-type allele, although SNP-wise it is distinguishable from the others. Exons (gray boxes) are segments of a gene that encode for the protein to be made. Introns are the intervening sequences between exons that often have no known specific function. A SNP in an intron is likely to have no effect, whereas a SNP in the regulatory or coding sequences (exons) may have a profound dysfunctional effect.

sequences. Essentially, all these loci are marked locations in the genome that can be detected as "SNP tagged" DNA segments. We next generate the SNP profile on all 400 loci in 25 members of our study family, look at the overall "SNP read-out," and search for patterns. Realize we do not yet know anything about these genes, but for convenience I have already called them Normal Lipids Gene A, etc.

One approach used for this sort of study, the "affected sibpair" approach, examines the SNP profile of the 400 loci to see which SNP alleles are shared between siblings who both have elevated cholesterol and triglycerides. If there are loci tagged by the same SNP in sibs who also both had hyperlipidemia, this might indicate something useful. This approach works on the assumptions that we have no expected number of genes involved, we do not know how much environment plays into the disease process, and we do not expect that every heterozygous or homozygous person will definitely show the disease. In genetics jargon this is called a "model-free" or "nonparametric" method of study (Nussbaum, McInnes, and Willard 2001).

As our gene hunt proceeds, a couple of interesting patterns show up (Table 11.3). Remember that I have simplified the data for demonstration, since the analysis originally started out with 400 loci identified by two SNP alleles each. Note that Locus A SNP 2 and Locus D SNP 2 are most often found in the individuals who have the worst lipid profiles. There are some exceptions. Sally

Table 11.3. A SNP profile of four loci analyzed in a sample of family members

Family members	Locus A	Locus B	Locus C	Locus D	Blood lipids	
					TC	TG
Robert	2/2	2/1	1/1	2/1	⇑	⇑
Dorothy	2/1	1/1	2/1	2/2	⇑	N
Andrew	2/2	1/1	2/1	2/1	⇑	⇑
Sally	1/1	2/2	1/1	2/1	N	N
Eric	1/1	2/2	2/2	1/1	⇓	⇑
Lara	1/1	1/1	1/1	2/1	N	⇑
Doug	2/1	2/1	2/1	1/1	N	⇑
Michele	2/2	2/2	2/2	2/2	⇑	⇑
Paul	2/1	2/2	1/1	2/2	⇑	⇑
JoAnn	1/1	1/1	1/1	1/1	N	N
Miriam	2/2	2/2	2/1	2/1	⇑	⇑
Margaret	1/1	1/1	2/1	2/1	⇑	⇓

Note: TC, total cholesterol; TG, triglycerides; N, normal.

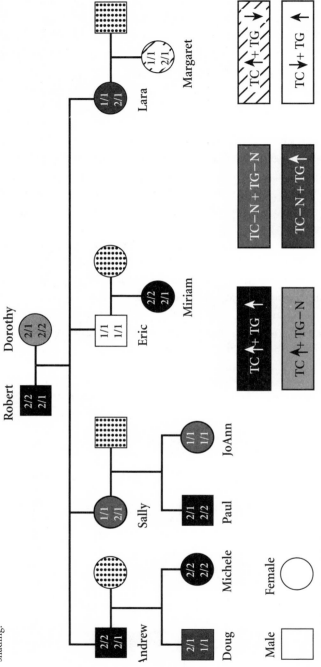

Figure 11.3. Genotypes representing the alleles shown in Table 11.3 for Locus A (top set of number) and Locus D (bottom). Total cholesterol (TC) and triglyceride (TG) phenotypes are shown. Relative changes are displayed as high (↑↑), normal (N), and low (↓). Combinations are coded by shading.

(Locus D—2/1) has normal lipids, Eric (Locus A—1/1; Locus D—1/1) has elevated triglycerides, and Margaret (Locus D—2/1) has low triglycerides. In actual studies there are also exceptions. This is why a large number people with clearly defined phenotype measures such as blood lipid concentrations provide the strongest data. We know nothing about what functions the loci or genes represented here may have, or even if we should suspect them to be involved in lipid metabolism. Even if the people were not related, we could look for an association of Locus A (allele 2) or Locus D (allele 2) with elevated blood lipids. We would want to compare similar genetic analyses on a control population that does not show lipid abnormalities. We could then calculate an odds ratio as to the likelihood these loci are associated with elevated lipids. This finding would not prove cause and effect, only indicate that this locus should be studied in more detail.

Illustrated in Table 11.3 is a simple profile of alleles (alleles 1 or 2) at four "demonstration" loci (A, B, C, D). This family has had a continuous history of hyperlipidemia through the generations. The numbers shown in each column refer to which SNP was identified at each locus for each person. For example, Robert inherited a SNP allele 2 at Locus A from both his mother and father. Note that SNP 2 alleles for both Locus A and Locus D tend to show up in individuals who also have elevated blood cholesterol or triglycerides or both.

Another factor that I have not displayed here but is essential in the sibpair analysis is the pedigree relationship of these people. Table 11.3 shows data on individuals with no particular inheritance relationships. Knowing that an allele will be passed from one generation to another allows us to calculate its predictable occurrence. Therefore, we can test these calculated or predicted probabilities with our actual observations. A statistical calculation can be made to test the hypothesis that a particular SNP allele and the lipid abnormality have a relationship. This statistical evaluation would tell us whether the suspected relationship was simply occurring by a lucky chance. The evaluation, made by calculation of a maximum likelihood odds ratio, tests the possibility that the allele sharing in affected sibs has a greater likelihood than the 50% possibility that this result occurred by chance.

In order to get a statistically strong result, we would need many more people involved in this study than those shown in Figure 11.3. In Figure 11.3, Locus A alleles and Locus D alleles are shown along with the phenotypes of total cholesterol (TC) and triglycerides (TG). We would also want to investigate other families to make sure that the set of alleles found in this particular study is not unique to this family. If our search revealed new genes that influence lipid metabolism, even if only in this family, we have discovered another important part of the puzzle. We would hope that these genes are important in a wide segment of the population.

Tracking Disease with SNPs

We must now prove that these two SNP alleles influence lipid metabolism. We could go into the human genome database and find out what is already known about the region of DNA surrounding the SNP identified in our study. Is this SNP related to any previously identified gene? Is the SNP in some functionally relevant part of a gene, like a coding region or a regulatory region? Could the SNP be the actual disease-causing mutation or is it simply a "marker" of a locus that is tightly linked to some other change in an important gene close by? Some of the answers to these questions can be pursued by simply studying the DNA segment in question. We could have selected the original 400 SNPs for this analysis to reside within intragenic regions, thus increasing the possibility that the SNP variation may represent functional differences. For example, there are computer programs that can detect what are called "open reading frames" of DNA sequence. These frames indicate regions that are highly likely to encode for protein rather than serve as noncoding regions or possibly "junk" DNA. Coding regions are characterized by a three-nucleotide code (triplet code) of sequences that must be strung together side by side for a long distance and that must make "coding sense," and these features are detectable by computer searches. Therefore, if a region truly is an open reading frame, we should be able to decipher the DNA sequence and clearly read it off, with no mistakes, as an amino acid sequence making up part of a protein. If the SNP of interest resides within this coding stretch of sequence (Figure 11.2, Allele 2) and introduces an error in how the triplet code is interpreted, then we may have discovered a disease-causing mutation. Another functional disturbance induced by the SNP might be a regulatory one (Figure 11.2, Allele 3). A SNP disturbing the coding sequence is relatively easy to figure out because open reading frames are not hard to spot, and a disrupted amino acid sequence is functionally easier to explain than a putative regulatory sequence mutation.

Compared with coding sequences, the sequences that govern gene regulation and the overall level of expression are less strict (conserved). These regulatory regions of genes contain sequences that respond to activation or inactivation by transcription factors. They often have certain sequence patterns, but they commonly have minor sequence differences that are hard to predict without functional studies. Transcription factors are proteins that regulate gene expression via specific interactions with DNA regions where the promoter and enhancer sequences reside. A functional consequence is that the SNP has disrupted a regulatory sequence that is important in turning a gene on or off at the proper time (Figure 11.2, Allele 3). Frequently, either hormones or a buildup or deficiency of metabolites finely regulates many genes involved in lipid metabolism. Many hormones, like insulin and glucagon, function by turning genes either on or off. For example, insulin frequently turns genes on for lipid synthesis during "times of plenty." Insulin works through a complex set of signals that eventually activate gene transcription. During gene transcription, the DNA sequence is converted into an RNA copy. The RNA, in the form of messenger RNA (mRNA), is then "translated": a protein is synthesized by the assembly of amino acids in the order dictated by the triplet code of the mRNA, which originated from the DNA sequence of the gene. If a SNP occurs that alters the structure of the protein made from the mRNA, that change can be detected. If the SNP is outside a reading frame, it is much trickier to determine whether it has any functional significance. It could be junk DNA and have no functional significance whatsoever. It could be in one of the regions between coding segments (Figure 11.2, Allele 4), again without necessarily affecting gene function.

Now back to our SNP. Let's say that the SNP resides in a sequence that is critical for regulating transcription of the gene of interest. Recall that glucagon is often the opposing hormone to insulin. So when it's time to turn down fatty acid synthesis, the insulin concentration should decrease while the glucagon concentration rises. In normal circumstances this should turn off the fatty acid synthesis genes. This turn-off process may require interactions now by another transcription factor inducing a signal event. Only this time, this event is induced by glucagon at a different site in the regulatory region of this gene. For our example, let's say that the region of DNA that responds to insulin signaling is wild-type or normal, but the segment of DNA that should respond to glucagon is interrupted by the SNP we are tracking. The functional result is that insulin can turn the gene on at the appropriate time, but glucagon cannot fully signal it to turn off at the appropriate time. So in this example, a SNP induces a change in a gene that has nothing abnormal at all in its coding region. This gene makes a perfectly normal enzyme that produces fatty acids profusely, but it won't turn off properly when the glucagon signal arrives—the SNP has disrupted its response element. A person with a SNP in this position would have this fatty acid synthesis gene allele always on, or activated, and would have hypertriglyceridemia.

What I have so far described is hypothetical. We have only been playing with DNA sequence data; we have not done any real functional studies. A few critical things remain to be done before launching into functional studies of this SNP locus. It would be useful to know if this particular SNP is found widely in the population or if it is a "private polymorphism" limited to a single family, and if it seems to show up most frequently in people with lipid abnormalities. Answering these questions may be tricky, because we most frequently found (Table 11.3) this SNP (Gene A, allele 2) in combination with another one (Gene D, allele 2). It may be that in order for it to have an effect, it must co-occur with the other one. In complex diseases, like lipid disorders, there may also be a functional requirement for the right combination of dozens of gene variants, identifiable by SNP analysis, for the clinical phenotype to appear. Any other combination, short of this "magic combination," will not result in a lipid disorder because the net effect is below clinical threshold, the gene-environment tipping point. Contrast this situation with the much less common situation of familial hypercholesterolemia, where all that is needed is a single mutant allele in the LDL-receptor gene and disease will occur. SNP tracking is simply a method of tagging DNA segments in the genome that allows researchers to track down genes that may influence disease processes, such as those of lipid metabolism.

SNPs and Drug Function

There is a great deal of interest in this SNP business, coming not only from scientists trying to identify the genetic basis of disease but also from the pharmaceutical industry. Pharmaceutical companies are extremely interested in finding SNPs that would predict the best effects of their drugs in patients (Roses 2000). They seem most interested in SNPs that may predict undesired side effects or toxicities in patients who might take their drugs. Imagine this scenario: A patient goes to see his physician, who decides the patient needs drug X for his high blood triglycerides. The doctor takes a blood sample and performs a quick SNP analysis of the DNA found in his white blood cells. She determines from the profile of 20 different SNPs that drug X works 87% of the time, but the profile of 14 other SNPs tells her that drug X has a 35% chance of causing liver toxicity in patients with these 14 SNPs. Of course, this story ignores any environmental effects, such as other drugs currently being taken, diet, or activity, and other major influences on lipid metabolism, like age. From a purely genetic point of view, information like this would be extremely valuable to many pharmaceutical companies; therefore, some companies have invested heavily in the human genome project. This area of medicine is called pharmacogenetics. It is just one aspect of what geneticists envision as individualized genetic (single genes) and genomic (many genes in combination) medicine of the future.

I want to leave you with one final note about SNP hunting. Although this is undeniably a powerful approach for following many genes among people, many geneticists, including those in pharmaceutical companies, have great hopes for this technology to discern not only the many genes involved in causing complex traits like lipid disorders, but also the genes that are influenced by drugs. There is significant skepticism among other geneticists, however, as to the power of this or maybe any genomic approach to bring to our attention the potentially large number of individually variable genes that make up a complicated disease with fairly subtle, highly variable clinical differences. Remember, cloning the gene for cystic fibrosis was an enormous task, but it was comparatively easy because mutations in this one gene result in a single disease. In contrast, a patient with complex lipid disorders may not only need to have a collection of several specific alleles of many genes that provide minor modifications of the lipid profile, but also to have all or most of them occurring together in order to produce a discernible phenotype. Metabolic diseases are further complicated by major influences from sex, ancestry, diet, and activity level.

Individualized Genomic Medicine

I have described in this chapter diseases with a complex causal development. The different genes involved can be searched for using SNPs as "ID tags" of genes to follow through families and entire populations. Researchers try to find highly reproducible patterns of disease traits that occur at the same time as certain SNP-tagged alleles of putative disease-associated genes. Geneticists can then eventually clone the gene involved and test the functional status of that particular allele. Finally, if we were able to put together all of this genetic information on an individual, future patients may benefit from a complete genomic read-out of the possible alleles of genes known to influence the development of diseases. This genomic read-out will have to be considered, together with the person's lifestyle and environmental influences, in any assessment of his or her possible disease risks. This combined genetic and environmental assessment may also help both patient and doctor know whether a given drug may help a particular condition or have harmful side effects. Of course, a downside to having all of this potentially useful information is that others could abuse it, such as life insurance companies who will only insure people with certain "low-risk" genetic characteristics. In contrast, a major positive outcome to these genetic studies will be the revelation of new disease mechanisms that will point researchers and doctors toward new disease prevention measures, and new drugs that we have not even considered before. It remains to be seen whether a broad genomic read-out as envisioned here is technically possible at a reasonable price and is as informative as we expect.

Parts I and II of this book have covered the basics: where fat comes from, how it is burned, and what is known about the genetic components that contribute to both single-gene disorders of lipid metabolism and the multifactorial basis of a person's net lipid phenotype. In the next section I will apply this information to an exploration of ways to maintain or improve a person's net lipid phenotype.

PART III

Knowledge into Practice

CHAPTER 12

Overcoming Genetics and Aging

The processes involved in the development of diseases of excess fat are complex, and so are the solutions. The unalterable factors of genetics and the aging process may also add to the challenge of remaining lean and healthy. To prevail over genetics and aging, one must understand what *can* be changed—nutrition, both the quality and quantity of foods consumed; activity level; and, possibly, drug intervention. Many aspects of our environment and behavior should be examined for solutions. Furthermore, we must recognize that all people are different, and no one solution fits all.

Genetics and the Environment

Even the fittest of us notice a tendency, as we age, to gain weight in the midsection and have higher blood cholesterol values—this pattern of change is influenced both by the genes we inherited from our parents and by the aging process. As an introduction to this section of the book, in this chapter I discuss the influence of our genetic heritage along with the aging process on body fat phenotype. Our genetics and aging, neither of which we can change, can be positively influenced by things we can control, such as diet, exercise, and if necessary, drugs.

Many of us can identify with Pam's situation (see box). She is in middle age and has a busy schedule with many demands placed on her time. In the coming decade, Pam will have the additional major life change of menopause, which will markedly influence her body fat phenotype and risk of long-term disease. We do not know other specific disease risks from Pam's genetic history beyond the fact that her mother has diabetes. There is a good chance Pam also has a predisposition toward diabetes as she reaches her older years.

In some populations, such as the Pima Indians of Arizona (Gila River Indian Community), the genetic predisposition for development of obesity and type 2 diabetes is unusually high (Baier and Hanson 2004). I will use this group to illustrate how ancestry (or genotype, the genes one inherits) can have a marked effect on phenotype (one's physical characteristics) while at the same time the environment has great influence on phenotype as well. The good news is we can often change our environment.

The Pima Indians living south of Phoenix, Arizona, have been studied intensively since 1965 to understand their high prevalence of obesity and type 2 diabetes. The ancestors of this group are believed to have lived in this area for over 2,000 years, although diabetes as a major health problem has only appeared during the twentieth century (Knowler et al. 1990). The Pimas had successfully adapted to desert life by irrigation farming (50–60% food supply), fulfilling the remainder of their food needs with indigenous plants, seeds, and animals. This all changed when European settlers arrived in the area. First, arrival of the new immigrants led to diversion of the Pimas' irrigation water supply, which changed their farming practices. Second, the new social and environmental conditions led to lifestyle changes, such as the purchase of food rather than the production of it and the availability of foods different from those in their traditional diet. By 1969, traditional dishes were prepared only

---

A Common Scenario

Pam is accompanying her 76-year-old mother, Sara, to the doctor for treatment of diabetes and other weight-related health problems. At 43, Pam's body is starting to thicken around the waist and she's gained seven pounds since her last annual physical. As her own preteen kids get older, she finds herself spending more time chauffeuring them to activities and sports instead of getting exercise herself. And she is relying more often on convenience foods to get meals on the table because of the family's hectic schedule. What can she do to prevent herself from acquiring the apple figure and attendant health problems she is now witnessing in her mother?

on special occasions, and the Pimas had adopted the average United States diet (Knowler et al. 1990).

In many ways the Pimas' development of diet- and activity-related health problems, such as obesity, diabetes, and cardiovascular diseases, is similar to the experience of peoples who have immigrated to the United States from India, Japan, and China and subsequently consumed a western diet. These immigrants develop the same health problems as seen in the Pimas, whereas people with similar genetic inheritances who remained in their homelands, consuming their traditional diets, have fewer of these disease problems.

The Pimas appear to be especially predisposed genetically to these health problems. Perhaps their successful adaptation to desert life over millennia was supported by genetic adaptations that, in an environment with a readily available food supply, can only be considered an unfortunate combination. The Pimas of Arizona have a natural "control group": a population descended from the same ancestors but who live in a remote mountainous location in northwestern Mexico and follow the traditional lifestyle lived by the Arizona group in earlier centuries. The prevalence of obesity and diabetes in the Mexican Pimas is much lower than that seen in the Arizona group, although they are genetically very similar (Ravussin et al. 1994). The experience of the Arizona Pimas is an example of what can happen when a genetically stable population encounters a rapid change in environment. In this case, it revealed a group of people very sensitive to excess calories and reduced activity.

Menopause Changes and Other Effects of Aging

As women approach fifty years of age, they begin experiencing the changes of menopause. This "change of life" has many hormonal effects that affect the body fat phenotype. It is not unusual for women to maintain premenopausal body *weight* but to lose lean body mass and muscle mass while gaining total body fat, especially visceral or abdominal fat (Lee, Kasa-Vuba, and Supiano 2004). That is, the body fat distribution pattern changes from one resembling a pear to one resembling an apple. This means increased visceral fat and its subsequent problems when present in excess, particularly the tendency toward developing insulin resistance and worsening blood lipid profiles. Loss of the sex steroids contributes substantially to a rise in total cholesterol, LDL cholesterol, and triglyceride concentrations in the blood (Nerbrand et al. 2004).

As both men and women age, there is an overall reduction in our capacity to oxidize fat and glucose because of reductions in mitochondrial oxidative and phosphorylation processes (Petersen et al. 2003). This facilitates the development of insulin resistance. In studies performed on healthy, lean (BMI < 25), sedentary, elderly (ages 61–84; male and female) individuals matched with healthy, young (ages 18–39 years; male and female), lean (BMI < 25), sedentary individuals, it was found that mitochondrial function was markedly lower (-40%) in the older subjects than in the young controls (Petersen et al. 2003). The elderly group had elevated blood glucose and insulin values during a glucose tolerance test, and with further testing the elderly group was also found to be significantly insulin resistant and to have more lipid stored in their muscle and liver tissues. Even in lean, healthy individuals, then, there develops a tendency toward insulin resistance. Of course, obesity would further aggravate the normal aging process. Positive actions, such as resistance training, that help improve this situation will be discussed in Chapter 14.

The Challenge to Change

If the goal for an individual is to prevent or reduce excess body fat and reduce risk of disease, there are several things to consider. The obvious ones are always diet and exercise practices. There are also less obvious considerations, such as an individual's overall attitude about life and how it might affect his or her eating and exercising practices. Psychological factors are involved in all of healing, including fat loss and disease reversal; however, I will not discuss these factors in any detail. For example, there is a well-studied psychology of binge eating after dieting and stress and this has been modeled in rats (Hagan et al. 2002). Furthermore, there is a complex relationship between obesity and depression, one that is difficult to sort out. Are people obese because they are depressed or are they depressed because they are obese?

Eating Styles versus Fad Diets

Conditions of excess fat can be dealt with on several fronts that in many cases require overcoming genetics and aging. The most obvious challenge is at the level of calories in and calories out. Controlling incoming calories is most effective because exercising away excess fat is not nearly as efficient. For most people it is easier to not eat a sugary, high-fat cheesecake dessert worth 800 calories than to exercise away the same number of calories with 1–2 hours of fairly vigorous exercise (see Table 14.1). Therefore, in order to control calorie intake for the long term, a new way of eating must be established. There is an overabundance of diets out there, all claiming to have the secret of successful weight loss. Most have some basis for working and probably have worked for someone, somewhere, for at least a few weeks. There are many excuses for going back to one's old ways. There are many excuses for a diet that didn't work: it was complicated—too many things to count, keep track of, or trade; it required that strange, expensive, and unsatisfactory foods be substituted for familiar ones; it didn't satisfy hunger pangs most of the time; and it required discipline. It's pretty clear over the long term; diets do not work most of the time.

Perhaps what is required is a new way of eating, an "eating style," considered part of a lifestyle, with quantity a major focal point rather than exactly what kind of "diet" it is as far as "high this" and "low that." The important question is this: what eating style will (a) provide a balanced diet of palatable and varied foods so that the plan is easy and enjoyable to follow, (b) reduce hunger and provide mental and physical fuel throughout the day, and (c) work well with the patient's lifestyle and time constraints to balance calories in with energy out? If a person can identify that type of eating style, then that person has made the most important step in reducing excess body fat—that is, finding the most effective ways to reduce caloric intake. It is probably more important to reduce overall calories than to get terribly uptight about exactly what the foods are that make up the diet, assuming the diet provides balanced nutrition and the required vitamins, minerals, essential amino acids and fatty acids, and fiber. Many experts have their own opinions on what is the ultimate, best diet, but most diets have no long-term studies to support claims beyond short-term weight loss. That is, virtually none have long-term research to show that it reduced disease and increased life span. I don't believe there is such a thing as the ultimate, best, one diet fits all.

In 1995 the Baby Boom generation turned 50, and the generational waistline has expanded along with the years. Over the past twenty years a plethora of diets have earned favor, ranging from extremely low fat to the long popular high-protein, high-fat Atkins diet. I will cover the Atkins diet in some detail in the next chapter. Unfortunately, a great deal of confusion has been generated over the decades because at times we were told not to worry about the carbohydrates but to avoid fat at all costs. At other times, we were told to avoid carbohydrates and not to worry about fat. Despite this confusion, I don't think anyone would argue that high-calorie meals, high in both fats and carbohydrates, are the worst combination. The arguments arise when we debate the most effective means of reducing calorie intake. Clearly, gram for gram, fats have twice the calories of carbohydrates. Strictly from that perspective, it makes sense to reduce dietary fat. Carbohydrates, however, turn into fat and stimulate insulin secretion; in excess, they too constitute a high-calorie meal. Furthermore, when some fats—such as *trans* fats, which currently seem to be ubiquitous in commercially prepared foods—are combined with sugars and starch (as in many fast-food meals), they increase risk of cardiovascular disease independent of obesity. Therefore, whether one eats more carbohydrates or more fat, the calories in, calories out balance is a given. Different people will have different responses to dietary fat and carbohydrates, yet whatever their response is, all must find the way to match calorie intake to energy expenditure. Patients who need to lose excess fat will only be successful when they find an eating style that allows them to eat things they like, that is not too complicated, or that doesn't require ingredients that are hard to get. Most important, their eating style must satisfy their hunger, or they won't tolerate it for long.

Exercise

Everyone needs to exercise on a regular basis to keep the fatty acid burning system well tuned. Choosing an exercise program is like choosing an eating style; it must work for the individual. Finding exercise that can be done with minimal hassle is a key factor. Some find if they can slip into their exercise shorts and shoes and take off out the door, they will exercise on a regular basis. If they have to drive to an exercise facility, change clothes, wait for exercise machines, and so on, they won't do it. Others, however, like the companionship of the exercise club and can't wait to get there every morning. If so, then they have found their way to a successful exercise regimen over the long term. Doing different exercises as schedules permit breaks up the monotony of doing the same thing everyday. Exercise needs to be appropriate for the stage of life. For example, pounding the payment or the basketball court may not be the best exercise for some, especially those with bad knees, whereas swimming or bicycling may be better for them. The main point here is that everyone needs to find enjoyable activities, decide where they most like doing these activities, and make it convenient enough that they will participate on a regular basis. (see Chapter 14 for a more detailed discussion of exercise.)

We will all be better off if we can find a way to eat and a way to exercise that keeps our weight down. We need to find a way to reduce calorie intake by reducing hunger and to choose a diet that promotes for burning of fat rather than making and storing more fat (see Chapter 13). We also need to find an exercise routine (Chapter 14) that we will do daily and perhaps even miss if we miss a day. Clinical observation and research both suggest that the way to long-term weight maintenance is making lasting changes in eating patterns rather than going on and off a series of restrictive diets. I believe this approach will help everyone to be on the road to a long-term lifestyle that will reduce excess body fat and improve health status, as well as to feel terrific physically and mentally. It is better to discover a new way of eating that matches calorie expenditure and provides adequate nutrition than to be "on a diet" of some sort. The goal is a long-term, healthy lifestyle rather than a quick diet or the latest exercise craze.

Sometimes Drugs Are Required

Many clinicians prefer to get blood lipids under control and increase insulin sensitivity through lifestyle changes, but when these strategies fail new drug options may help. Some drugs are very effective at helping reverse conditions of excess fat. Some are definitely more effective than anything we can do by diet or exercise. I believe we must use these medicines when needed. It is preferable to try lifestyle changes first and to continue that strategy even if drugs are required later in addition. Unfortunately, none of the prescription weight-loss drugs are approved for long-term use; they are intended for short-term weight loss, not lifelong weight maintenance. The mechanisms by which some of these drugs work are discussed in Chapter 15.

Signs of Progress

Anyone trying to eat and exercise optimally to lose fat and increase muscle mass will naturally want to see results. There are some simple ways to evaluate progress. The bathroom scale is the first line of evaluation. It is best to keep to a consistent time of the day for weighing, such as early morning before any food or drink is taken. Body weight fluctuates 2–3 pounds because of hydration status without any changes in fat or muscle mass. The goal is to have the same baseline body conditions, as described, to obtain the best weight measurement for evaluating progress.

Furthermore, the goal is fat loss, not weight loss. Doctors recommend that dieters preserve or increase muscle mass. Some individuals may reach a point where they are adding muscle mass, losing fat, yet gaining weight. Muscle bulk is heavier than fat bulk, so this scenario is possible, especially among those who exercise a lot. Unfortunately, the bathroom scale will not distinguish fat loss from water loss or muscle gain. It takes sophisticated instruments—such as dual-energy x-ray absorptiometry, CAT scanning, or other body imaging techniques—to evaluate body fat and lean mass. Obviously, these measures are only taken in special circumstances, such as research studies or detailed evaluation for other purposes. Insurance will not pay for most individuals to have their body fat and lean mass determined under ordinary circumstances.

Another simple estimate of visceral fat loss is measuring waist and hip circumferences. The ratio of waist-to-hip circumference is used to monitor visceral obesity. This is a fairly crude estimate that may be informative for following an individual's changes, rather than trying to use certain ranges for evaluation. A person with an apple or android shape (and a high waist-to-hip ratio) who loses body fat may reduce waist circumference and the reduction in waist-to-hip ratio demonstrates improvement. On the other hand, this will not be as useful for a person with a pear or gynoid shape and predominantly excess peripheral fat. People with a normal BMI and no excess visceral fat have waist-to-hip ratios in the range of 0.7–0.9, whereas those with BMI values in the obese range characterized by visceral obesity may have values greater than 1.0 (Wang et al. 2005). These measurements for a given individual can be followed over time to monitor improvements in visceral fat reduction. Following waist circumference alone, as I described as one of the criteria of metabolic syndrome (Table 5.1), may be more predictive (Wang et al. 2005) of risk for development of type 2 diabetes.

Another sign of success is simply feeling better. Carrying around less weight is more comfortable. Leaner people are more encouraged to take the stairs instead of waiting for the elevator. Once they start feeling slim, with more energy and much less hunger, dieters will be very encouraged to continue their new lifestyle. A simple thing like bending over to pick up something from the floor is a breeze. It may even feel good to stretch those muscles.

If drugs are required, physicians will usually employ more sophisticated measures of success, such as evaluations of blood lipids, glucose, insulin, and other metabolites and hormones. Sometimes it is necessary to measure liver or muscle enzymes, because some drugs have side-effects that may damage these organs. One way to evaluate these effects is to measure enzymes that leak out of cells when they are injured by the drugs. These are rare side-effects, but they do occur. The hope is that, as body fat reduces, blood lipids, glucose, and insulin values will do likewise. Over time, these values should return to the normal range.

To reach and maintain a healthy weight, people should find an eating style that offers adequate nutrition and that includes foods they enjoy, and most of all reduces their hunger. Next, it is helpful to find an exercise routine that will be done on a regular basis, as well as other activities that are enjoyable and burn calories. Many clinicians reserve drugs for people with conditions resistant to change by lifestyle modification, but recommend that lifestyle changes be made anyway.

In this section of the book I will build on the overall discussion started with this chapter. The goal is to demonstrate how the knowledge gained from the earlier sections can be used to reverse or prevent the diseases of excess fat. Next, I turn our focus to the possibility of breaking the insulin cycle.

CHAPTER 13

Breaking the Insulin Cycle

Some believe that low-fat diets—that is, diets made up of high-carbohydrate foods—are automatically low in calories and guaranteed to help reduce body fat. This is not true, however, because excessive carbohydrates, like all excess calories, will also turn into fat. This chapter explains how low-fat, high-carbo-hydrate diets may severely affect the body's fat metabolism, especially for those who already are insulin resistant. Diets high in sugars and starch not only provide the starting material or substrate to make excess fat, but they also may not contain enough healthy fats to signal a shutdown of fat synthesis and stimulate fat burning. Excessive insulin secretion is an important component in insulin resistance. There are major benefits to disrupting the vicious cycle of excess insulin production. This chapter also explains how low-carbohydrate diets, such as the Atkins diet, seem to work, although we lack enough infor-mation to assess the long-term effectiveness and safety of these relatively high-fat diets. It will also discuss the controversy over the glycemic index and put into perspective debates over the health effects of both fast foods and low-fat foods.

The Low-Fat Gospel

For many years, low-fat, high carbohydrate diets were the gospel for weight loss and health promotion. The benefits of a diet low in saturated fats were first recognized back in the 1960s with the Seven Countries Study led by Ancel

Keys. This study showed that there was an association between saturated fat in the diet and heart disease; however, as pointed out by Walter Willett, the study did not find any connection between total dietary fat and heart disease (Willett 2001). Beyond these findings with regard to saturated fat, the low-fat gospel has been preached ever since. The U.S. Department of Agriculture (USDA) regularly published the well-known "Food Guide Pyramid" promoting this idea that maintaining health requires consuming a low-fat diet. The American Heart Association, American Cancer Society, and the World Health Organization all supported the concept for many years. In recent times, however, this certainty has come into question. The issue of low-fat, high-carbohydrate vs. high-fat, low-carbohydrate diets has become a focal point of debate as to the possible causes of the current epidemic of obesity, insulin resistance, and diabetes. Articles in popular magazines and the professional press provide an abundance of debate on these dietary approaches (Taubes 2001; Bray 2003; Ornish 2004; Willett 2004). One thing everyone can agree on is that the current state of affairs—with so many people consuming an excess of calories from both fats and carbohydrates—is a complete disaster.

If total calories are kept constant, however, are there differences in the health effects between a diet high in fat and one high in carbohydrates? Studies are currently being done to answer this question, often with surprising results. During a recent experiment in my lab, for example, the results were so unexpected that our first response was, "We must have mixed up the blood samples." How could we find higher blood triglycerides in the mice that ate the low-fat, high-carbohydrate diet than in those who ate the high-fat diet? In this experiment my research student, David Kurtz, and I were studying the effect of a high-fat diet on mice that had a genetic deficiency in the enzyme long-chain acyl-CoA dehydrogenase (LCAD), which is required for mitochondrial fatty acid oxidation (described in Chapters 9 and 10). David was testing the hypothesis that a genetic deficiency of fatty acid oxidation, which causes elevation of free fatty acids in blood, would make mice prone to insulin resistance and obesity (Wood et al. 2003). In other words, we postulated that if the mice can't burn fat, they will store fat. David did the study with what we jokingly called our "McDonald's diet," made with beef tallow (beef fat—relatively high in saturated fat) to have over 40% of calories from fats. The standard mouse diet in the laboratory setting is often only 10–12% fat. For this experiment, we needed a control diet (low-fat diet for comparison) with the same calorie density, or calories per weight of food. This meant we needed a diet that was high in carbohydrates, rather than high in fat. We made up the needed calories with starch. So the experiment was essentially done as a high-fat versus a high-carbohydrate diet experiment.

We found some surprising results, one of which was that the mice that ate the high-carbohydrate diet developed hypertriglyceridemia. Among the mice eating the high-carbohydrate diet, the LCAD-deficient males had the most pronounced hypertriglyceridemia, followed by the normal males. Next were the LCAD-deficient females, and the normal females had the lowest blood triglycerides. In contrast, regardless of whether or not they had LCAD deficiency, all of the mice that ate the high-fat diet had normal blood triglycerides. Again, this was such a surprising result to me that I thought we had the blood samples switched, so we checked everything, and the results were correct. The low-fat, high-carbohydrate diet induced hypertriglyceridemia in these mice; it was most severe in the mice that had the genetic deficiency of fatty acid oxidation when controlling for sex, and most severe in the males. What was going on here?

As a metabolic geneticist, these results were a paradox to me. That is, if an individual has a genetic deficiency in the ability to burn fat, a high-fat diet should make the blood fat increase—right?—but it was the high-carbohydrate diet that did so. Fortunately, I have some colleagues in nutrition who pointed out that this sort of thing happens in people too. Some investigators consider elevated triglyceride concentrations as an important independent risk factor for cardiovascular disease, more so in women than men (Austin 1999). I had also been very curious about the fact that Americans were buying more and more low-fat to no-fat foods but were on average becoming more obese and more insulin resistant all of the time. There seemed to be an association between increasing consumption of high-carbohydrate, low-fat foods and more people developing insulin resistance, type 2 diabetes, and obesity. This presumed association, however, does not prove that high-carbohydrate, low-fat foods cause insulin resistance, diabetes, and obesity. In light of our surprise results in the mouse experiment, however, it all looked very curious to me.

The paradox intensified when Walter Willett, from the Harvard School of Public Health, gave a seminar at our university on November 6, 1998. He talked about the negative effects of eating less fat in our diets and said we needed to increase our intake of polyunsaturated and monounsaturated fats, an argument he later made in his book (Willett 2001). He strongly recommended that we should be using regular salad dressings with the full allotment of soybean or olive oils and that we should eat more nuts. He said that eating high-carbohydrate diets at the expense of fats, especially healthy fats like monounsaturated and polyunsaturated fats, was associated with several diseases. I thought, "What is this guy saying? Everyone knows we should eat low-fat diets!" Dr. Willett, however, is a highly regarded authority concerning the effects of diet on health, and he showed compelling data to support his claims. Furthermore, there were those nagging results we found in our mice.

About this time, I met a medical student who came to me after my biochemistry lecture on lipid metabolism. He had previously experienced dangerously high blood triglycerides and cholesterol, and had gone on the Sugar Busters diet (Steward et al. 1995). As a result, he lost some weight and reduced his blood lipids. Of course a high-fat diet, like Sugar Busters, is heresy to the standard low-fat, high-carbohydrate diet gospel.

Sugar Busters is based on the premise that protein and fat should be substituted for carbohydrates. The entire thesis of Sugar Busters is that carbohydrates in the diet, especially those with high glycemic indexes (to be explained a little later), promote for excessive insulin secretion and, in turn, insulin promotes excessive fat synthesis. In many ways, the thesis of Sugar Busters concerning carbohydrates and excessive insulin secretion made sense to me.

One key issue in the Sugar Busters approach was the claim that protein does not promote for insulin secretion as sugar does. Gerald Reaven, whom we met in Chapter 5, has contributed a great deal to our understanding of insulin resistance (Reaven, 1988). Dr. Reaven is another early proponent of a relatively low-carbohydrate diet for treatment of insulin resistance, but he does not promote the idea of replacing so much carbohydrate with protein and saturated fat (Reaven, Strom, and Fox 2000). There are, however, many anecdotal accounts of people who lost weight and improved their blood lipids while following Sugar Busters. For various reasons, however, many who tried this diet did not stick with it over a long time period. The story told by the medical student, however, added to my curiosity about the idea that excess calories from low-fat, high-carbohydrate foods may be no more healthy than excess calories from fat and carbohydrates.

The Atkins Diet

The Atkins diet is the antithesis of the low-fat, high-carbohydrate diet (Atkins 2002, 2003). This diet was developed by the late Robert Atkins in the early 1970s. Although it was the predecessor to Sugar Busters and other low-carbohydrate diets, the original low-carbohydrate diet is credited to William

Banting (1796–1878), whose *Letter on Corpulence Addressed to the Public* was published in 1863. (Do not confuse William Banting with Frederick G. Banting, one of the discoverers of insulin.) The controversy of the Atkins diet is that it is a high-fat and high-protein diet, and it has the *reputation* of consisting exclusively of bacon, eggs, and steaks while its adherents lose weight and lower blood lipids. The key questions are: How can this be? How safe and effective is this diet?

The concept behind the Atkins diet is that by going through four phases, the body's metabolism changes from principally carbohydrate utilization and fat storage to predominantly fat burning (Atkins 2002). The first and most drastic stage of the diet, induction phase, is when total carbohydrate intake is limited to less than 20 grams per day. The dieter is supposed to eat meat and eggs until "satisfied" but not "stuffed." Induction is the period of most weight loss. During the next three phases, low-carbohydrate vegetables and fruits are gradually added to the diet, yet total carbohydrate intake remains limited to maintain both reduced hunger and the desired body weight.

Apparently, many people lose significant weight during this first phase, as they do on many diets when they actually monitor, at least temporarily, what they are eating. Clinical trials using low-carbohydrate diets have now demonstrated this (Samaha et al. 2003; Foster et al. 2003; Brehm et al. 2003; Stern et. al. 2004; Yancy et al. 2004). The presumed reason is that reduced carbohydrate-stimulated secretion of insulin helps stabilize blood glucose concentrations and this, in turn, reduces hunger. Reducing insulin also reduces insulin-promoted fat synthesis from carbohydrates and reignites fat burning. So although individuals on this diet may be eating more fat and protein, the net effect is that they are eating fewer calories because they are not as hungry. At the same time, this approach promotes fat burning instead of fat storing. Dr. Atkins's book describes monitoring this fat-burning process by evaluating the development of ketosis. Ketosis is an elevation of ketone bodies in the blood. Ketones are produced during fat burning, so someone in ketosis is definitely burning fat, which requires insulin to be low. Note well: ketosis is not the same as life-threatening ketoacidosis, which develops in type 1 diabetes patients.

Despite what I have seen written many times, apparently by writers who have not experienced this approach, the reduction in appetite is not a result of chronic nausea. As Dr. Atkins described in his books, during the first 2–3 days individuals may feel a little weak in the stomach, as the body switches from excessive carbohydrate use to predominantly fat burning for fuel, but that soon dissipates. Beyond those first couple of days, most people seem to feel fine and enjoy being less hungry. There do not seem to be clear data explaining the mechanism of reduced hunger. Many assume that it involves the reduction in the overall insulin secreted (because of lower carbohydrate ingestion) and avoidance of hypoglycemia-induced hunger. Others believe it is an effect of the ketosis. I have not found any convincing data demonstrating either mechanism, and in certain experimental situations insulin has been demonstrated to act as an appetite suppressant.

My main concern about this diet is the relatively high saturated fat and cholesterol content. Reaven expressed the same concern in his book *Syndrome X* (Reaven, Strom, and Fox 2000). The trends I have seen from personal experiences and from various published studies indicate that what Dr. Atkins predicts seems to hold true for most people practicing this diet. He predicts that total blood cholesterol concentrations will decrease, as will triglycerides (assuming that blood is drawn after fasting, as is usually the case). LDL cholesterol will stay the same as it was or increase slightly and HDL cholesterol will tend to increase. These general trends have held up in the clinical trials mentioned above. Both higher HDL and lower triglycerides are desirable. I am still amazed, given all of our preconceived notions about dietary fat, that there is such a drastic weight loss in many people who try this approach, and that their blood lipids do tend to improve. One note of caution is that some individuals do respond with elevated blood lipids, thus monitoring blood lipids is probably a wise thing to do. Another point about blood lipid concentrations is that many people have lower lipids when they are losing weight and are in negative energy balance, whereas their lipids may not remain low after their weight stabilizes again. A final, often overlooked point about the blood lipid concentrations is that, regardless of what a person's dietary habits are, we usually do not know what the lipid values are following a meal. Since blood is drawn to determine lipid values usually after an overnight fast, even with a high-fat diet the lipid values may be low after a fast. Thus, the important unknown is the blood lipid concentrations following the meal, and this may pose an undetected lipid challenge to the body. I know of no direct long-term studies (a year or longer) investigating the cardiovascular effects of the Atkins or any other low-carbohydrate diet.

Reduced body fat and lower blood lipids all sound like good, short-term changes, but what we don't know yet are the long-term risks and benefits of this diet. Bravata and colleagues (2003) published a review from the literature of the studies published to date concerning low-carbohydrate diets. At that time, as summarized by Bray (2003), they concluded "that lower carbohydrate

Table 13.1. Carbohydrates, fat, and calories in three breakfast menus

Item	Quantity	Calories	Total fat (g)	Saturated fat (g)	Cholesterol (mg)	Protein (g)	Total carbs minus fiber: "impact carbs" (g)
Breakfast							
1 Banana	1	104	1	0.2	0	1	25
Cereal: Great Grains, with skim milk	1 cup each	480	9	0.5	0	8	70
Grapefruit juice	1 cup	100	0	0	0	1	24
Totals		684	10	0.7		10	119
Breakfast 2							
Banana	1	104	1	0.2	0	1	25
Fat-free yogurt	1 cup	120	0	0	5	12	19
Oats	0.5 cup	150	3	0.5	0	5	23
Cereal: Grapenuts	0.5 cup	250	1	0	0	6	42
Pineapple	1 serving	60	0	0	0	0	14
Totals		684	5	0.7	5	24	123
Breakfast 3							
Eggs	2	140	9	3	430	12	0
Bacon	4 slices	160	14	5	30	10	0
Totals		300	23	8	460	22	0

diets (< 60g/d carbohydrate) were associated with reduced calorie intake and that weight loss was predicted by calorie intake, diet duration, and baseline body weight, but not by carbohydrate content." In five recent studies comparing the Atkins diet or similar low-carbohydrate diets with low-fat diets, many obese subjects lost weight and improved their blood lipids (lowered triglycerides and raised HDL cholesterol) in the short term (6 months) on the low-carbohydrate diet more than those following a conventional low-fat diet. After a year, however, in many cases the initial weight losses were regained and body weights were almost equal between the two diet groups, because many of the subjects did not stick with any diet (Samaha et al. 2003; Foster et al. 2003; Brehm et al. 2003; Stern et al. 2004; Yancy et al. 2004). In all the studies compliance tended to be better with the low-carbohydrate diet. There were no major adverse effects reported in any of the studies. Compliance may be a key factor with any diet; diets are difficult for many people to stick with in the long term because they require discipline.

The Atkins diet is not quite the hedonistic indulgence many first think. Unfortunately, many followers and critics do not seem to get past the induction phase. This diet was not intended as a perpetual diet of bacon, eggs, and sausage with no fruits and vegetables. In fact, as adherents progress through the stages of the Atkins diet, their diet may eventually contain a large proportion of salads, fish, and low-starch fruits and vegetables (Atkins 2003). For whatever reason, I frequently hear that women have a more difficult time sticking with the Atkins diet than men. Furthermore, the diet requires exercise, too: Dr. Atkins entitled one section in his book "Exercise: It's non-negotiable" (Atkins 2002)! Modifications of the original Atkins low-carb approach have been made by Fred Pescatore, a former associate of Dr. Atkins in developing the Hamptons diet. He has emphasized less saturated fat and more monounsaturated fats, particularly from macadamia nut and olive oils—preferably those produced with minimal processing. A very interesting and unique contribution of his book is an appendix that explains the different types of dietary oils and how they are produced (Pescatore 2004).

I will demonstrate by using an example why I think the Atkins approach works for those who adhere to it. Table 13.1 describes three possible breakfasts. Breakfast 1 includes a whole-grain cereal with some added sugars, skim milk, fresh fruit, and unsweetened fruit juice. Breakfast 2 eliminates added sucrose (unsweetened, nonfat yogurt and added fruit and a cereal with no sugar added), but it is fairly low in total fat. Both breakfasts look "healthy" by traditional criteria; however, in my own experience hunger returns within an hour or two after both. Note in Table 13.1 the column listing total carbohydrates minus fiber, which gives an estimate of the "impact" carbs that seem to affect insulin and appetite.

In contrast, breakfast 3 has negligible carbohydrates, a high amount of fat—in particular, a relatively high percentage of saturated fat—but only half the total calories in the other two "healthy" breakfasts. The important difference is that hunger does not return for 4–5 hours after breakfast 3, rather than 1–2 hours. So the perceived low-carb advantage is that an individual starts off with half the calories and has no need for a snack within 1–2 hours. I believe this is the key to the low-carbohydrate approach. Thus, overall it would appear that the Atkins diet is a high-fat, lower-calorie diet because of the reduced intake of carbohydrates. In other words, the diet reduces the perpetual appetite that carbohydrates purportedly stimulate via insulin secretion via rising and falling blood glucose concentrations, as well as many other mechanisms researchers do not fully understand yet. This concept was further supported by a clinical trial in obese patients with diabetes (Boden et al. 2005), which leads us directly into the whole issue of the glycemic index.

The Glycemic Index

Another part of this paradox—that low-fat, high-carbohydrate diets may be associated with increased obesity—fell into place when I heard about the *glycemic index* of foods. This is an index relating how quickly and how high different foods raise a person's blood glucose after eating them. The glycemic index is determined in people by measuring blood glucose concentrations following ingestion of the test food and comparing them with the concentration following ingestion of the reference food (Foster-Powell, Holt, and Brand-Miller 2002). A value of 100 is assigned to the response obtained from the standard reference foods, which are 50 grams of glucose or consumption of white bread containing 50 grams of carbohydrate. Carbohydrates include common sugars (Table 13.2) as well as the complex carbohydrates, predominantly starches like the ones in potatoes, and fiber. To keep things simple, I will refer to these different carbohydrates as sugars, starches, or fiber.

Starches are long molecules made up of many glucoses attached to one another. They may have branching patterns that affect their digestibility. The long-held assumption was that starches took longer to digest and would raise blood glucose concentrations more slowly than pure sucrose ingestion. It turned out, however, that white bread was as quick a source of blood glucose as pure sucrose. Since people are more willing to eat bread than an equivalent amount of pure glucose, white bread has become a common reference food for this test.

There have been suggestions that reducing the intake of foods with a high glycemic index may help regulate blood lipid concentrations and also manage diabetes, as well as prevent the development of insulin resistance and cardio-vascular disease. Although this sounds like a reasonable possibility, large clinical studies to make us confident of these benefits are still lacking.

Another possible factor in using the glycemic index is appetite control. Maybe you have noticed that after eating a high-sugar meal, like traditional pancakes with syrup, you may feel "stuffed" but it won't be very long before you are feeling hungry again. Eating foods with a high glycemic index—thus raising blood glucose concentration quickly and quite high, with a responding insulin secretion and subsequent blood glucose lowering—may cause this feeling of hunger. It has been assumed that the pancreas quickly and vigorously responds to an increase in blood glucose with a strong output of insulin. Insulin secretion first causes blood glucose not only to go down, but also to drop below normal. The result is a feeling of hunger. This has been described as "food-driven insulin stimulation and reactive hypoglycemia." Although I have heard even some famous diet doctors describe this, I've been unable to find convincing data that reactive hypoglycemia actually occurs in most people. Hunger pangs are caused by a complex set of events, including low blood glucose, that trigger a signal in the brain that it is time to eat again.

Several important concepts emerge from these observations about the glycemic index. As alluded to earlier, most everyone, including researchers and dieters, assumed that starches were slowly digested and released sugar components gradually, unlike the sharp spike of blood glucose that occurs when people eat straight sugar. It was clear from the data obtained by determining the

Table 13.2. Common sugars

Common name	Sugar constituents	Common sources
Glucose	Glucose	Breakdown of sucrose and starch
Fructose	Fructose	High-fructose corn syrup, fruits, and breakdown of sucrose
Sucrose	Glucose + fructose	Table sugar
Maltose	Glucose + glucose	Beer
Lactose	Galactose + glucose	Milk

glycemic index, however, that many of the starchy foods caused a spike in the blood glucose peak, just as the sugars did. For example, if bread equals 100, table sugar (sucrose) has a glycemic index of 97, ten jelly beans equals 82, and a baked potato has an index of 121. Baked potatoes are usually on everyone's list of healthy high-carbohydrate foods, but according to their glycemic index they are worse than pure sugar as far as raising blood glucose concentrations. Carrots are often pointed out as being surprisingly high in the glycemic index range; however, a wide range of values have been reported for carrots. Carrots are a good example of the need to consider the *glycemic load* of foods. The glycemic load is the glycemic index multiplied by the quantity of carbohydrate being eaten. As Willett points out in his excellent book, *Eat, Drink, and Be Healthy*, in order to get the effect used to establish the glycemic index, 50 grams worth of carbohydrate, a person has to eat 1.5 pounds of carrots (Willett 2001). In the amounts usually eaten, carrots have a pretty low impact. How foods are cooked also affects their glycemic index. For example, look at potatoes baked (121) versus boiled (80–124) in Table 13.3. Also, all starches are not equal. Depending on the nature of their molecular structure, they may or may not break down quickly to raise blood glucose concentrations. This is determined by the ratio of two substances contained in a carbohydrate molecule, amylose and amylopectin. Amylose is slower to digest than amylopectin. Amylose is higher, for example, in legumes such as beans. This ratio explains some of the differences in glycemic index and how cooking may also have a significant effect. Fiber is essentially indigestible by humans and does not raise blood glucose concentrations.

The glycemic index is still controversial with many skeptics (Pi-Sunyer 2002), although there appears to be increasing agreement about the benefits of

Table 13.3. Glycemic index (GI) values of common foods (numbers based on white bread as the standard)

High-glycemic foods	GI values	Lower-glycemic foods	GI values
White bread (standard)	100	Oat bran (50%) bread	63
Cooked potatoes (baked)	121	Cooked potatoes (boiled)	80–124
Orange juice	74	Orange	60
Banana	74	Apple	52
Table sugar	97	Peanuts	21
Pancake (no syrup)	96–146	All-Bran cereal (Kellogg's, USA)	54
Carrot (boiled)	46–131	Carrot (raw)	23

Note: Values are from Foster-Powell, Holt, and Brand-Miller (2002).

controlling glycemic index and load in health maintenance, especially in regard to diabetes patients (Sheard et al. 2004). The American Diabetes Association has not accepted glycemic index for recommendation for use by diabetes patients, however. Some of the difficulties with the glycemic index are that it is complicated to use with good predictability, because factors such as ripeness of fruits, size of foods when cut and cooked for serving, cooking methods, and many other variables markedly affect the glycemic index or glycemic load predictions (Pi-Sunyer 2002). Many of the existing studies done to establish the glycemic indexes used isolated foods (i.e., all carrots, all potatoes), but people don't eat single food items; they eat a mixture of things that add fat, protein, and especially fiber, which appears to be an important variable as to how fast carbohydrates are absorbed after eating. It remains to be seen whether the glycemic index or glycemic load turns out to be a practical and useful measure in developing and following diets. Further research is under way to validate more fully the usefulness, as well as the practical limitations, of the glycemic index and load in dietary management (Brand-Miller et al. 2003). Regardless of the remaining difficulties, the work done to investigate glycemic index and glycemic load has changed our understanding of complex carbohydrate dynamics, especially of starch, in ways that may be important in controlling the problems of insulin resistance, diabetes, and obesity. Specifically, it has corrected the assumption that starchy foods release their sugar content slowly; in fact, many starches are actually digested fairly quickly and raise blood glucose and insulin levels. Again, like the mice in our experiment, people who eat foods with a high glycemic index, especially those who are already insulin resistant, also often have higher blood triglyceride concentrations. People who have metabolic syndrome and high blood triglyceride concentrations also tend to have especially small, dense LDL particles in their blood. Many investigators believe that small, dense LDL particles more readily undergo oxidative modification, thus contributing to the development of atherosclerotic lesions. It is important to point out, therefore, that low-fat, high-carbohydrate diets also tend to be diets with a high glycemic load and that this may help perpetuate the vicious insulin cycle.

Dietary Carbohydrates and High Blood Lipids

A growing body of data from studies done in both animal models and in people indicate that many lipid diseases may not be helped by a low-fat, high-carbohydrate diet as previously assumed. It seems logical that individuals who eat less fat should have less fat in their body, be it in the blood or in the adipose tissue stores. Excess fat is caused by excess intake of calories from fat, carbohydrate, or protein. My point is that a low-fat diet may not be a low-calorie diet, nor must a high-fat diet be high in calories. Just because a food was not ingested as fat does not mean it cannot turn into fat. Thus, an excessive intake of low-fat, high-carbohydrate foods can set the optimal situation to produce body fat, even if fat is not taken in via the diet. My thesis is that low-fat, high-carbohydrate foods in excess, via insulin stimulation, promote for endogenous fatty acid and triglyceride synthesis in liver and inhibit fatty acid oxidation in muscle, whereas, calorie for calorie, fat would not stimulate insulin secretion. Insulin is a storage hormone. It promotes fatty acid synthesis and storage and inhibits fat burning. Insulin-resistant individuals, who already have compensatory hyperinsulinemia, may benefit by reducing their carbohydrate-driven insulin secretion (Reaven, Strom, and Fox 2000). Having excess calories, even from carbohydrates, in turn stimulates a double effect of expediting the development of hypertriglyceridemia and elevated free fatty acids in the blood. Both high triglycerides in tissues and elevated fatty acids in the blood and tissues seem to be the causes of, or at least markers for, development of insulin resistance and eventually diabetes, along with a high risk for cardiovascular disease. Of course, the caveat is that dietary fat in excess will also be stored. An underlying contemporary problem with the human body, which is perpetuated by our genetics, is that it evolved to be extremely proficient at energy storage because that mode of operation was required for survival in much earlier times, before the current ready supply of food. Our environment has changed from scarcity to abundance, but our bodies are still programmed to hoard calories.

Excess carbohydrates stimulate increased fatty acid synthesis by providing abundant substrate (generation of acetyl-CoA via glucose oxidation) and the stimulus (insulin) for fatty acid synthesis. Malonyl-CoA and acetyl-CoA (Chapter 8) increase after blood glucose and insulin concentrations rise, setting the stage for increased synthesis of fatty acids and triglycerides. The opposite, but beneficial, effect is that if carbohydrates are replaced by fat in the diet, particularly unsaturated fatty acids, these fatty acids will naturally tend to suppress the body's own synthesis of fatty acids: the body would "sense" that enough fat has come in from the diet. So on a low-fat, high-carbohydrate diet, the body thinks it is low on fat, and now it has plenty of carbohydrate substrate and insulin to get busy making fatty acids. After being synthesized, fatty acids simply don't hang around; they will be combined with a glycerol and made into triglycerides. Triglycerides will be stored, pathologically, either in tissues such as liver or muscle or an expanding adipose tissue. The excess triglyceride in the liver will be exported as triglyceride-rich VLDLs and promote for a higher concentration of atherogenic, small, dense LDLs. Of course, simply adding fat to a high-carbohydrate diet is the worst option, because now the body has a carbohydrate-induced insulin signal not only to *not* burn fat but also to make and store more fat, including the dietary fat. This is insulin resistance in the making!

The process of carbohydrate-induced fatty acid synthesis resulting in hypertriglyceridemia is complex, and many studies have been done in humans (Hudgins et al. 1996, 2000). Some interesting trends have come out of these studies, although all the results are not completely clear. Many of the human studies have been done with purified foods taken in liquid and solid form, which are not regular foodstuffs. Furthermore, there has been a wide range of results in the people studied (Parks and Hellerstein 2000). Overall, the trend has been for an increased concentration of blood triglycerides in most people who previously ate a moderate- to high-fat diet and then switched to a low-fat, high-carbohydrate diet. For some people, the change may be a transient one, and their blood triglycerides may go back down to baseline concentration after a few weeks (Parks and Hellerstein 2000). It appears that sugars were the worst at driving the increase in blood triglycerides, and of the sugars, fructose was the strongest offender. Sugars ingested in liquid form with no fiber, like in soft drinks, stimulated hypertriglyceridemia the most. Take a look at the first and second ingredients on the labels of carbonated soft drinks. First, you will find carbonated water, and second is high-fructose corn syrup (56% fructose). The consumption of high-fructose corn syrup in the United States has been increasing rapidly over the past 30 years—the same period that has witnessed an increasing prevalence of obesity and diabetes, especially in children (Ludwig, Peterson, and Gortmaker 2001; Bray, Nielsen, and Popkin 2004). In 1970 the estimated average intake of high-fructose corn syrup was virtually none; by 1980 it had reached ~27 grams/day; by 1990, ~70 grams/day; and by 2000, ~90 grams/day (Bray, Nielsen, and Popkin 2004). Therefore, I speculate that sweetened soft drinks are the perfect substrate for carbohydrate-induced hypertriglyceridemia, as well as obesity. Today these drinks seem to be a food staple for children and adults alike. The fiber contained in foods is beneficial, and this is why whole fruits containing fructose are milder offenders along these lines. The calorie content of two medium apples is equal to a 12-ounce soft drink. Which is more readily consumed?

Humans Synthesize Fat from Carbohydrate

Some very convincing studies have shown that when humans were fed iso-caloric (equal-calorie) diets of 10% of calories from fat and 75% from glucose versus diets of 40% of calories from fat and 45% from glucose, for 25 days, fatty acid synthesis was higher with the low-fat diet (Hudgins et al. 1996). On day 10 of the study, there was a markedly greater pool of endogenously synthesized palmitate ($C_{16:0}$-saturated fatty acid) in the VLDLs of the people on the high-carbohydrate diet than in those who ate the same amount of calories but with a diet containing fat. In contrast, fatty acid synthesis was minimal in the people eating the diet with fat. Another key point here is that endogenous synthesis promotes for a high proportion of the less desirable saturated fatty acids, such as palmitate, whereas dietary fats can be the more healthy ones, such as the mono- or polyunsaturated fats, especially the long-chain omega-3 fatty acids, which mammals are unable to synthesize. So not only did this study show an increase in fatty acid synthesis per se, but it also showed an increasing amount of the unhealthy saturated fatty acids resulting from endogenous synthesis. Further studies by these investigators also showed that these effects occurred whether the people were lean, obese, or diabetic (Hudgins et al. 2000). Palmitate ($C_{16:0}$) seems to be a particularly offensive saturated fatty acid as far as disease risk. In contrast, many studies have shown that another saturated fatty acid, stearate ($C_{18:0}$), appears basically neutral with regard to increased disease risks, but it has weak to virtually no positive effects like those for the long-chain omega-3 fatty acids.

I am not proposing that dietary fats are nowhere to be found in the body after being consumed. The concept here is that excess carbohydrates promote for excess insulin release, aggravating the situation in those already hyper-insulinemic, and insulin promotes for fat synthesis. Excess carbohydrates are a ready substrate for fatty acid synthesis and fat storage. Consuming excess fat will also add to the fat depots of the body. Fats in the diet are sometimes more subtle than realized, but they still add up. The blatant ones are cream, butter, and fatty meats, but less obvious ones include oils, some of which are *trans* fats, for frying or salad dressings. Also overlooked constituent oils include those found in avocados, nuts, seeds, and deep-water fish. Therefore, consuming excess calories as sugars and starch along with excess fat is the ultimate bad combination. Furthermore, counteracting these effects in practice means focusing on both the *kind* of carbohydrates—for example, selecting high-quality carbohydrates (legumes, whole grains, and fiber, with minimal processing) in place of sugar and highly processed starch—and the *quantity* (portion control).

The other side of the coin is that we can find mechanisms that explain the benefits of some dietary fats—especially the unsaturated variety. The important net effect will be a lack of insulin response along with promotion of fatty acid oxidation (as is seen when patients with hypertriglyceridemia are given a fibrate drug; see Chapter 15) and a reduction in fatty acid synthesis via mechanisms that also involve unsaturated fatty acids. In the next section I move on to these molecular mechanisms and explain how healthy fats may counteract the actions of too much insulin.

Molecular Mechanisms Promoting Fatty Acid Oxidation

As I will describe in the exercise chapter (Chapter 14), vigorous aerobic exercise sends a strong signal via epinephrine to burn fat for energy expenditure, and during exercise insulin is low and not promoting for fatty acid synthesis. Another mechanism considered pivotal in stimulating fatty acid oxidation and reducing VLDL secretion of formed triglyceride in the liver is the peroxisomal-proliferator activated receptor (PPAR) mechanism. Several pieces of evidence suggest the importance of this mechanism, though I must admit that direct human data are lacking. Let me make the case, however, because the evidence from studies in rodents is pretty good. The three major PPARs are PPAR-α, PPAR-γ, and the recently recognized PPAR-δ (Kersten, Desvergne, and Wahli 2000). (I will discuss PPAR-γ further in Chapter 15.)

The PPARs are *ligand-activated transcription factors* that are "switched on" by a variety of long-chain unsaturated fatty acids and fatty acid–related metabolites, which are low in high-carbohydrate, low-fat diets. A transcription factor is a special protein that is activated by another molecule (the ligand), such as a fatty acid. When a transcription factor is activated in the cell nucleus, it turns on a gene or genes so that they perform whatever function they have. They might, for example, increase the level of mitochondrial enzymes needed for increasing fatty acid oxidation. This is another example of the mechanism described in the discussion of SREBP regulation of cholesterol synthesis, back in Chapter 4. Natural ligands that activate PPARs and fatty acid oxidation include polyunsaturated fatty acids (PUFAs). That is, there are some dietary fatty acids that appear to activate fatty acid oxidation. In general, fatty acids with longer chain lengths and unsaturation status (i.e., the number of double bonds) are more potent for stimulating fatty acid oxidation via activation of

PPAR-α. Thus, fish oils containing the omega-3 fatty acids eicosapentaenoic acid (EPA, or $C_{20:5}$) or docosahexaenoic acid (DHA, or $C_{22:6}$) are most effective (Neschen et al. 2002). These oils are useful for lowering blood triglycerides, via mechanisms I will describe next, and they are cardioprotective.

My thesis is that diets rich in long-chain polyunsaturated fatty acids—that is, omega-3 fatty acids—may stimulate fatty acid oxidation, whereas diets rich in simple carbohydrates may stimulate fatty acid synthesis and inhibit fatty acid oxidation via promotion of malonyl-CoA synthesis. In contrast to omega-3 fatty acids, PPAR-α binds with lower binding affinity to saturated C_{18} fatty acid, which is also known as stearic acid ($C_{18:0}$), and to the monounsaturated fatty acid oleic acid ($C_{18:1}$). PPAR-α is found primarily in tissues that rely upon fatty acid oxidation for energy production—liver, heart, skeletal muscle, and kidney. Moreover, PPAR-α mediates the effects of peroxisomal-proliferator drugs of the fibrate group, like gemfibrozil (Chapter 15). Therefore, fibrates have frequently been used for treating hypertriglyceridemia and they appear to affect human hypertriglyceridemia by increasing fatty acid oxidation and decreasing secretion of VLDL. Note that it is the unsaturated fatty acids that activate PPAR-α, which in turn promote for increased fatty acid oxidation and decreased VLDL-triglycerides. So this is a system whereby unsaturated fatty acids on the rise could stimulate their own oxidation. Fat builds up in the blood and the adipose tissues if the body's chemistry is not providing the strongest signal. Since saturated fatty acids are a weaker signal, a high-fat diet containing predominantly saturated fatty acids may be a weaker stimulant to promote for increased fatty acid oxidation.

Signal to Reduce Fatty Acid Synthesis

Unsaturated fatty acids also act as a signal to turn down fatty acid synthesis. Fatty acid synthesis is regulated by several mechanisms. One key mechanism is the transcription factor known as SREBP, which I described for regulation of cholesterol synthesis. Recall from Chapter 4 that SREBP-2 is the transcription factor that turns up cholesterol synthesis when it "senses" that cholesterol is low. SREBP-1 appears to work in a similar fashion: when fatty acids are low yet insulin and acetyl-CoAs are readily available, as after a high-carbohydrate meal, all systems are go for fatty acid synthesis, and SREBP-1 is the ringleader for stimulating this process. It turns out that polyunsaturated fatty acids promote for reduction of SREBP-1, thus turning down fatty acid synthesis

(Clarke 2001). That's good news: unsaturated fatty acids help to turn down fatty acid synthesis.

In summary to this point, lowering calorie intake and increasing energy output (activity level) may promote two major benefits: increased fatty acid oxidation and reduced stimulation of fatty acid synthesis. Excess calories from fat or carbohydrates can be turned into stored body fat. Reducing calorie intake and substituting some healthy fats (unsaturated fats, especially omega-3 fatty acids) in place of sugars and starch may help break what I have called the insulin cycle in insulin-resistant people with hyperinsulinemia. Not all people respond equally to the signals of high carbohydrates or high unsaturated fats. There is no "one size fits all" perfect diet. The only consistent prediction is that taking in fewer calories and expending more calories will result in body fat loss.

Reduced Fat Synthesis and Increased Fat Burning Promotes for Leanness

Drug studies and research in genetics also point to the mechanisms that I have described as diet-driven excessive fat synthesis with depressed fat burning. Although I have spent the past 15 years working on the perils of deficient fatty acid oxidation, I am now convinced that aberrant fatty acid synthesis—at least partially stimulated by excessive carbohydrates, and in addition to excessive fat intake—is a major factor in the epidemic of insulin resistance, diabetes, and obesity that we now see in the United States. Again, some experiments using mice, in which profound effects were observed when fatty acid synthesis was reduced, either genetically or by experimental drug treatments, have had a great influence on my thinking.

The first example is that of a drug that inhibits an enzyme called fatty acid synthase. Fatty acid synthase is essential for building fatty acids from the carbohydrate sources of acetyl-CoA and malonyl-CoA (Chapter 8). Mice given the compound known as C75 showed a 95% reduction in fatty acid synthesis from acetyl-CoA (Loftus et al. 2000). These mice had profound weight loss. They also drastically reduced their food intake, so the C75 reduced not only their fatty acid synthesis but also their calorie intake. There is also a genetic example of what happens if individuals cannot synthesize triglycerides completely. Mice with a genetic deficiency of an enzyme known as acyl:diacylglycerol transferase remain very lean even when fed a high-carbohydrate diet (Smith et al. 2000). These mutant mice demonstrated that disrupting the process of storing fatty acids as triglycerides also promoted for leanness. They simply cannot make the normal amount of triglycerides. You may wonder where the free fatty acids end up if they cannot be incorporated into triglycerides. No one seems to know yet, but it may be that when fatty acids are high, a signal is received that says to not make more.

One other mouse mutant also gives us a strong indication of how accelerated fatty acid oxidation appears to decrease susceptibility to development of insulin resistance and obesity. This mouse has a mutation in the acetyl-CoA carboxylase-2 (ACC-2) gene (Abu-Elheiga et al. 2001). This is the mitochondrial form of the enzyme that makes malonyl-CoA. I have mentioned malonyl-CoA several times as the precursor of fatty acid synthesis and as the inhibitor of fatty acid oxidation at the carnitine palmitoyltransferase-1 (CPT-1) step. The CPT-1 enzyme, you may recall from Chapter 9, is the "gatekeeper" of fatty acid oxidation. So as it turns out, when ACC-2 is deficient, resulting in no inhibitory malonyl-CoA being produced, then mitochondrial fatty acid oxidation is unrestricted, working all the time—even when it would normally be inhibited by high insulin and all the signals to store fat rather than burn fat. As you can readily envision, these mice remain lean despite being fed all they want to eat.

Thus, what we find from the mouse studies is that mice given a fatty acid synthase inhibitor remain lean and reduce their food intake, and mice with a genetic defect in triglyceride synthesis at the step of adding on the last fatty acid to a diacylglycerol remain lean. In the last example, if there is a genetic defect that takes the brakes off mitochondrial fatty acid oxidation, those mice remain lean. It appears from these different examples that animals remain lean either by reducing the ability to synthesize fatty acids and triglycerides or by increasing fatty acid oxidation. Furthermore, I would speculate that all of these lean mice have high insulin sensitivity.

A Comparison of Dietary Constituents in Different Diets

It is important to realize that a calorie is always a calorie. If we take in calories as fat, as sugar, as protein, or as alcohol, they will either be expended by energy output or be stored as fat or glycogen. When I am contrasting low-fat diets, with high amounts of carbohydrates, with those that have some unsaturated fat, I am assuming that both diets have the same number of calories, that is, they are isocaloric. In other words, I am not proposing that anyone eat more calories by adding healthy fat. I am suggesting replacement of an equal number of calories, or even reducing calorie intake, by substituting some of the carbohydrate components (sugars and starch) with some monounsaturated and polyunsaturated fats (Figure 13.1), as recommended by the Syndrome X diet (Reaven, Strom, and Fox 2000). This will likely be done by using vegetable oils rich in monounsaturated and polyunsaturated fats to avoid excessive saturated fat.

I was curious as to the fat and carbohydrate constituents of two diets, so I have devised a sample menu for a fast-food diet and a low-fat, high-carbohydrate diet to examine these factors (Tables 13.4–5). I went to the web sites of the companies listed or looked on food packages to obtain the calorie information shown. Furthermore, in Figure 13.1, I have shown the calculated body weight of a person who eats a specified number of calories, depending also on their level of physical activity, as determined for three different diets.

Most tables of nutritional content use the simple conversion factors of 9 calories for 1 gram of fat and 4 calories for 1 gram of both carbohydrates and protein. I calculated the calories on the basis of the more accurate numbers 9.3 kcal (1 kcal = 1 diet calorie) per gram of fat, 4.1 kcal/gram carbohydrate, 4.0 kcal/gram protein, and 7.1 kcal/gram alcohol. The companies that published the tables I consulted have also not included the amount of *trans* fat present in foods, which may be substantial; *trans* fats were reported as unsaturated fat. Certainly, one could choose different items and quantities of the foods listed in Tables 13.4 and 13.5, but I think each menu is a reasonable approximation of an average U.S. male's selections. Ironically, the fast-food diet is not far off from the percent distribution of calories in the categories of total fat, unsaturated fat, carbohydrates, and so on, recommended in the Syndrome X diet plan. The main problem is that there are way too many calories in the fast-food menu and likely a lot of hidden *trans* fat. I would emphasize again that what a person eats might be secondary to how much they eat. In the low-fat diet, there are fewer calories because calorie density of carbohydrates versus fats is around half. The caveat is the glycemic index effect of the carbohydrates and the potential stimulation of insulin secretion. This diet would be similar to the type of diet (high in starch) that caused hypertriglyceridemia in the mouse experiment I described in the beginning of this chapter. So lower calorie intake is certainly good, but an excessive insulin response may be detrimental. One eating strategy is to lower overall calories by including unsaturated fats as a replacement for sugars and starches, but not fiber. This type of diet should promote for fat burning and reduce fat synthesis. It also agrees

Table 13.4. A day's menus for a fast-food diet

Food	Calories	Total fat (g)	Fat calories	Saturated fat (g)	Saturated fat calories	Cholesterol (mg)	Total carbohydrates (g)	Carbohydrates (calories)	Sugars (g)	Protein (g)	Protein (calories)
Breakfast at McDonald's											
Sausage biscuit with egg	498	33	307	8	74	245	31	127	2	16	64
Hash brown potatoes	136	8	74	1.5	14	0	14	57	0	1	4
Orange juice	82	0	0	0	0	0	20	82	18	0	0
Totals	716	41	381	9.5	88	245	65	267	20	17	68
Lunch at Pizza Hut											
Breadsticks	131	4	37	1	9	0	20	82	1	3	12
Meatlover's pizza (2 slices)	658	34	316	14	131	60	56	230	4	28	112
Coke: supersize	463	0	0	0	0	0	113	463	113	0	0
Totals	1,252	38	353	15	140	60	189	775	118	31	124
Dinner at home											
Swanson Hungry Man XXL frozen dinner Backyard BBQ	1,161	48	446	18	167	225	110	451	72	66	264
Milo's Sweetened ice tea	172	0	0	0	0	0	42	172	36	0	0
Edwards Georgia pecan pie	444	20	186	4	37	30	60	246	34	3	12
Totals	1,778	68	632	22	205	255	212	869	142	69	276
Grand Totals	3,746	147	1,367	47	432	560	466	1,911	280	117	468
Total percent calories	100		36					51			12

Note: Values of nutrient components were obtained from each company's web site (McDonald's and Pizza Hut) or package label, and calories were calculated based on 9.3 calories/gram (fat), 4.1 calories/gram (carbohydrate), and 4.0 calories/gram (protein). Note 1 diet calorie = 1 kilocalorie.

Table 13.5. A day's menus for a low-fat diet

Food	Calories	Total fat (g)	Fat calories	Saturated fat (g)	Saturated fat calories	Cholesterol (mg)	Total carbohydrates (g)	Carbohydrates (calories)	Sugars (g)	Protein (g)	Protein (calories)
Breakfast											
Apple Jacks cereal	263	1	9.3	0	0	0	60	246	32	2	8
Barber's skimmed milk	89	0	0	0	0	5	13	53	13	9	36
Pop Tarts, grape frosted	206	5	47	1	9	0	37	152	18	2	8
Tropicana home-style orange juice	115	0	0	0	0	0	26	107	22	2	8
Midmorning snack											
Sara Lee bagel	250	0.5	5	0	0	0	50	205	5	10	40
Tropicana home-style orange juice	115	0	0	0	0	0	26	107	22	2	8
Morning Totals	1,083	6.5	60	1	9	5	212	869	112	27	108
Lunch											
Lean Cuisine glazed chicken	233	5	47	1	9	50	25	103	6	21	84
Snackwells devils' food fat-free dessert	53	0	0	0	0	0	12	49	7	1	4
Sugar-free Coca-Cola	0	0	0	0	0	0	0	0	0	0	0
Totals	286	5	47	1	9	50	37	152	13	22	88
Dinner											
Bud Light beer: 2	220	0	0	0	0	0	13.2	213[a]	0	1.8	7
Broiled chicken breast	123	2	19	0.5	5	65	0	0	0	26	104

Table 13.5 (continued)

Food	Calories	Total fat (g)	Fat calories	Saturated fat (g)	Saturated fat calories	Cholesterol (mg)	Total carbohydrates (g)	Carbohydrates (calories)	Sugars (g)	Protein (g)	Protein (calories)
Baked potato	123	0	0	0	0	0	26	107	3	4	16
Breakstone's fat-free sour cream: 2 tbsp	25	0	0	0	0	5	5	21	2	1	4
Del Monte whole kernel corn	62	1	9	0	0	0	11	45	7	2	8
Salad: lettuce, tomato, carrots	20	0	0	0	0	0	4	16	2	1	4
Kraft French fat-free salad dressing	45	0	0	0	0	0	11	45	5	0	0
French bread: 2 slices	136	1	9	0	0	0	26	107	2	5	20
Bluebell strawberry frozen nonfat yogurt	356	0	0	0	0	0	75	308	72	12	48
Bedtime snack											
Nabisco fat-free Fig Newtons: 4	188	0	0	0	0	0	44	180	22	2	8
Barber's skimmed milk	89	0	0	0	0	5	13	53	13	9	36
Evening Totals	1,386	4	37	0.5	5	75	228	1,095	128	64	255
Grand totals	2,711	16	144	2.5	23	130	477	2,115	253	113	451
Total percent calories	100	5		5			78				17

Note: Values of nutrient components were obtained from package labels, and calories were calculated based on 9.3 calories/gram (fat), 4.1 calories/gram (carbohydrate), and 4.0 calories/gram (protein). Note 1 diet calorie = 1 kilocalorie.
a. This value includes carbohydrate and alcohol calories.

with the positive effects found by Willett of having unsaturated fats in the diet (Willett 2001).

This chapter argued that excessive carbohydrates and low unsaturated fats in the diet (at least in some if not many individuals) stimulates excessive fatty acid synthesis and hence the development of hypertriglyceridemia and elevated free fatty acids, which in turn aggravate insulin resistance, if present, and probably facilitate development of obesity. Not everyone responds this way, but many do. Perhaps you find this conclusion—that a low-fat (but high-carbohydrate) diet may make a person fatter—as surprising as I did when I first began looking into the evidence. But, after all, the body has to put the newly synthesized fat somewhere.

I have explained how the glycemic index seems to be a possible indicator of which foods may provide a rapid source of blood glucose and raise insulin concentrations, which in turn raise malonyl-CoA concentrations that pro-

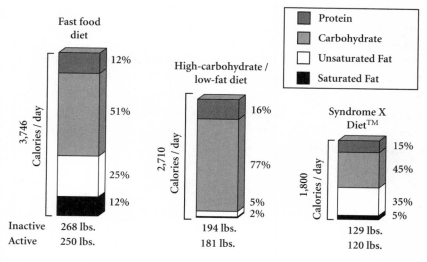

Figure 13.1. A graphical representation of calorie distribution and total calories of three possible diets. Menus for a fast-food diet are described in Table 13.4 and for a high-carbohydrate, low-fat diet in Table 13.5. Shown also are the body weights maintained by the caloric intake shown. These calculations were based on the formulas described in Reaven, Strom and Fox (2000).

mote for fatty acid synthesis. At the same time malonyl-CoAs are blocking the import of fatty acids into mitochondria for oxidation.

I have also described the beneficial metabolic effects of low-carbohydrate diets in mouse mutants. First, as in the lean ACC-2 mouse mutant, we humans can encourage fatty acid oxidation by exercising more and by reducing carbohydrate stimulation of ACC-2. This takes the malonyl-CoA "brakes" off of fatty acid oxidation. Increasing fat burning will help reduce blood triglyceride and fatty acid concentrations, thus reducing the potential for developing insulin resistance and obesity. Second, long-chain unsaturated fats, like omega-3 fatty acids, in the diet provide a stimulus via increased activity of PPAR-α for activating mitochondrial fatty acid oxidation while decreasing the activity of SREBP-1, which stimulates fatty acid synthesis when activated. Recall that drug inhibition of fatty acid synthase and the genetic defect of triglyceride synthesis were beneficial in promoting for leanness.

All these factors explain why a low-fat diet with high carbohydrate content may not be helping to control the epidemic of diabetes and obesity in this country. As I mentioned earlier, in many of the so-called low-fat packaged foods the fat is replaced by carbohydrates, often those with high glycemic indexes, such as simple sugars. Adding sugars to the diet is exactly what is *not* wanted for addressing the problems of diabetes and obesity. Finally, I agree with Dr. Reaven that syndrome X (metabolic syndrome) is a silent killer, but the risks can be reduced by reducing overall calorie intake, by substituting many of those carbohydrate calories, especially sugars and starch, with some unsaturated fat calories, and by burning off glucose and fatty acids through exercise. Exercise—a key ingredient in any diet or regimen for promoting health—is the subject we turn to in the next chapter.

CHAPTER 14

Exercise to Burn Fat

We all hear a lot about the benefits of exercise for weight control, stress relief, and overall physical health. But how exactly does exercise create these powerful changes in the body? In this chapter, I describe how anaerobic and aerobic exercise work at the cellular level and the impact this has on the body's energy balance and ultimately on weight loss or gain through the burning of stored fat in adipose tissue. I also discuss the improbability of a pill that would simply and safely burn off fat. Finally, I investigate the potential importance of using increased muscle mass as a way to burn calories without doing anything.

Different Muscle Types to Pump and Expend Energy

All activities, not only those we usually designate as exercise, contribute to the overall calorie burn throughout the day. Even standing burns calories, and many activities we take for granted or could easily add to our routine can make a significant contribution to the daily calorie expenditure. Our focus here will be exercise (both aerobic and anaerobic), muscle types (fast twitch and slow twitch, red muscle versus white muscle), and how to prevent or reverse insulin resistance. As described earlier, insulin resistance is defined as the requirement of abnormally higher amounts of insulin to get the same normal lowering of blood glucose concentrations. Exercise and development of insulin resistance are intimately tied to fat metabolism. At birth, less than 25% of the human body mass is muscle. This goes up to around 40% in young adulthood and drops back to around 30% in old age (Murray 2000). Thus, metabolic processes in muscle cells have a major impact on the net body metabolism throughout life. A muscle's metabolism can be adapted or changed, for better or worse, depending on the major uses required of it. A marathon runner (aerobic exerciser), sprinter (anaerobic exerciser), and couch potato (no exerciser) have different muscle metabolic characteristics. These characteristics are a function of training and genetics.

There are different types of muscle, and they have different metabolic characteristics. The muscle type of most interest here is striated muscle, which is the type of muscle used for moving the arms and legs and for breathing, as well as for pumping the heart. Under the microscope, cardiac muscle has much the same appearance as skeletal muscle from the leg. Since cardiac muscle is highly dependent on fatty acid oxidation, even at rest (80% of its energy), what I say about the metabolism of "exercise" also pertains to the simple act of breathing and pumping blood around the body. As far as exercise and whole-body metabolism are concerned, this discussion will concentrate on striated muscle.

Striated muscle cells are long cells with a complex set of internal filaments called actin and myosin. These filaments, upon an electrical signal from a nerve impulse combined with a supply of ATP energy, work together to make the muscle contract. The physical alignment of these filaments is what gives muscle its striated appearance. Striated skeletal muscle is further categorized as "red" or "white." Red muscle fibers, also known as slow-twitch or Type I fatigue-resistant muscle, are relatively loaded with mitochondria and myoglobin. Like hemoglobin in red blood cells, myoglobin is essential for transporting large quantities of oxygen, supplied by the blood, within the muscle cell for immediate use by the mitochondria during aerobic muscle metabolism. Red muscle, which is high in oxidative enzymes and less dependent on glycolytic enzymes, is the muscle designed for long-term energy expenditure. It is the red muscle mass that a marathon runner relies on for oxidizing fatty acids. In contrast, white muscle, also known as Type IIB fibers, is high in glycolytic enzymes but low in oxidative enzymes and has fewer mitochondria and less myoglobin. This type muscle depends mostly on the quick energy of the breakdown of glucose *(glycolysis)* and has no immediate need for oxygen or mitochondria. Its demands are like those of a sprinter—a quick burst of energy that need not last long. White muscle is also known as fast-twitch muscle. There is also a Type IIA, an intermediate-twitch muscle that is high in glycolytic enzymes and intermediate in oxidative enzymes. Human muscle mass is composed from all three types in approximately equal proportions. Examples of these muscle types include ocular muscles (fast-twitch, Type IIB), gastrocnemius muscle (Type IIA), and soleus muscle (slow-twitch, Type I). Sprinting and weight lifting use fast-twitch muscles, whereas long-distance running uses slow-twitch muscles.

A pound of fat has 3,500 kcal (diet calories). In order to lose one pound of fat, an individual would have to eat 350 fewer calories per day for ten days. What if that person wanted to eat the same number of calories, but burn off an extra 350 with exercise? That certainly is the other choice, but it takes a lot of exercise to burn off a pound of fat (see Table 14.1). A combination of lower calorie intake and higher calorie expenditure (exercise) is the optimal approach to weight loss. Heavier people burn more calories per activity, as shown in Table 14.1.

Even if weight loss does not occur after exercising, great benefits are gained by reactivating the body's muscles, cardiovascular system, and respiratory system. Exercise reduces the "couch potato" risk factor for cardiovascular disease, even without losing a pound. Of course, doing it once is not enough. Many recent studies investigating exercise and improvement of insulin resistance involved time periods of 4–6 months of regular exercise. These studies showed improvement with exercise alone, but the most favorable outcomes included both exercise and weight loss (Watkins et al. 2003).

Exercise has many effects on health. Overall, exercise will keep the muscle cells primed for energy production, which means burning both glucose and fatty acids. Muscle cells primed for energy production are also the muscle cells that maintain normal insulin sensitivity.

Anaerobic Metabolism

Muscular energy is fueled chiefly by glucose, fatty acids, or ketone bodies. Muscle has the capacity to store glucose in the form of glycogen. Under nor-

Table 14.1.   Energy expenditure per 60 minutes of activity

Activity	Kilocalories burned for body weight 150 lb / 200 lb	Activity	Kilocalories burned for body weight 150 lb / 200 lb
Bicycling 10–12 mph	408 / 546	Walking 3 mph	238 / 319
Gardening	340 / 455	Golf, carrying clubs	374 / 501
Tennis	476 / 637	Sitting quiet	68 / 91
Jogging	476 / 637	Standing	136 / 182

Note: Values based on calculations provided in Ainsworth et al. (1993); 1 kilocalorie = 1 diet calorie.

mal conditions muscle should not store fat. (The exception is in endurance athletes, who store some fat with no consequences for insulin sensitivity.) As muscle contracts, these fuels will be used either for quick and immediate energy or sustained energy needs.

First, I will describe glucose metabolism for muscle energy. After a person has eaten or during periods of rest, blood glucose is converted into glycogen, for storage in the tissues. Glycogen is like starch for animal cells. In the liver, glycogen is being "laid in" for future use during fasting for release into the blood to maintain blood glucose concentrations. In the muscle, however, it is being stored for the muscle's exclusive use when needed, as for a quick sprint. So what happens when we are ready for a sprint, be it an organized race or chasing the taxi with your briefcase in the backseat for three blocks? A bolus of epinephrine *(adrenaline)* is released from the adrenal medulla and the body is revved up for action, which takes energy. Epinephrine activates a pathway for turning on the enzymes in the muscle to start breaking down glycogen. The overall process of taking stored glucose as incorporated into glycogen and breaking it back down into free glucose for use by the body for glucose metabolism is shown in Figure 14.1. The enzyme *glycogen phosphorylase* is the major player turned on during this rush of epinephrine. Glycogen phosphorylase cleaves the bond between the glucoses attached to one another in the long strands of glycogen. Branches of molecules are bonded to these strands, and these bonds are broken by *debrancher enzyme*. Debrancher enzyme cannot do anything until after the longer straight strands are broken down, so activation of glycogen phosphorylase is key.

These enzymes break down the glycogen molecules into separate molecules of glucose. In muscle, the glucose remains and is reserved for use exclusively by the muscle cell where the glycogen was first located. The glucose is in the form of glucose-6-phosphate, and the attached phosphate makes the glucose unable to leave the cell: it must be used only in that muscle cell. In contrast, glycogen broken down in a liver cell can leave as free glucose, because the liver enzyme glucose-6-phosphatase frees it from the phosphate. The free glucose can leave the liver and go into the bloodstream.

If free glucose arrives inside a muscle cell by insulin-mediated uptake, as in the case of muscle receiving glucose from the blood, it is quickly phosphorylated into the glucose-6-phosphate form to trap it in the muscle cell.

During the next process, *glycolysis,* energy is extracted from glucose without using oxygen (the process is *anaerobic*). Glycolysis is known as anaerobic glucose metabolism and occurs in the cytosol, the fluid inside a cell. In contrast, aerobic metabolism, which requires oxygen, occurs in mitochondria. Glycolysis consists of a series of enzymatic steps that change one glucose molecule into two pyruvate molecules, two NADH+H$^+$ molecules, and two ATP molecules (Figure 14.1). ATP molecules are the main goal here, for these are the molecules that, by their breakdown, provide the cell with energy. If the conditions are anaerobic, the NADH+H$^+$ and pyruvate cannot go any further as far as energy generation. If oxygen is available and the pyruvate enters the mitochondrion, it is quickly converted into acetyl-CoA, like that also derived

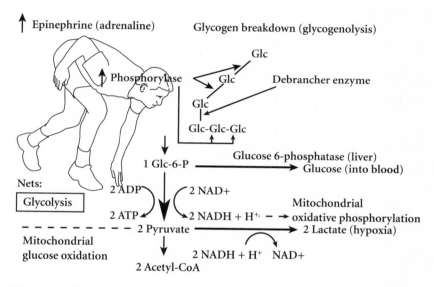

Figure 14.1. The transformation of glucose into energy. This pathway begins with the breakdown of glycogen, or glycogenolysis, which is initiated by an increase in epinephrine (here induced by exercise). Epinephrine activates the enzyme glycogen phosphorylase to break glycogen molecules down into glucose *(Glc)*. Debrancher enzyme detaches glucose molecules branching off from glycogen's main chain. Inside cells, the glucose molecules are phosphorylated into the form glucose-6-phosphate *(Glc-6-P)*, which cannot exit the cell. In hepatocytes, however, the enzyme glucose-6-phosphatase breaks off the phosphate and the resulting free glucose is able to leave the cell and enter the bloodstream. Glycolysis is the metabolic pathway that transforms Glc-6-P, ADP, and NAD+ into pyruvate, ATP, and NADH + H$^+$. If no oxygen is available, the pyruvate is converted into lactic acid, or lactate, and cannot be used for fuel. If oxygen is present, however, the pyruvate enters a mitochondrion and is converted into NAD and acetyl-CoA. Finally, the acetyl-CoA is used in the TCA cycle for production of energy as described in Chapter 9. Acetyl-CoA, acetyl coenzyme A; ADP, adenosine diphosphate; ATP, adenosine triphosphate; H, hydrogen; NAD, nicotinamide adenine dinucleotide; TCA, tricarboxylic acid.

from fatty acid oxidation. If oxygen is in short supply—because the person has been running a long time to catch a taxi, for example—the pyruvate is converted to lactate as a short-term trick to keep glycolysis going forward. This metabolic maneuver prevents the buildup of NADH+H$^+$ molecules by changing them back to NAD$^+$. Glycolysis will stop if the intracellular concentrations of pyruvate and NADH+H$^+$ molecules get too high and there are not enough NAD$^+$ molecules available. This is prevented by converting pyruvic acid (pyruvate) into lactic acid. The enzyme *lactate dehydrogenase* changes the pyruvate into lactate while also changing NADH+H$^+$ into NAD$^+$ to keep glycolysis going in the muscle (Figure 14.1). You may have heard of exercise-induced muscle cramps caused by the buildup of lactic acid. The lactic acid comes from these lactate molecules. This continues production of ATP in times of low oxygen or in cells that have no mitochondria, such as red blood cells. The bad news is that not a single molecule of fat has yet burned!

Phosphorylase breaks down the many glucoses of glycogen, and eventually the free glucose is phosphorylated to glucose-6-phosphate (Glc-6-P) to enter into the process of glycolysis (Figure 14.1). If glucose oxidation cannot proceed because of low oxygen, lactic acid builds up. If oxygen is available, pyruvate proceeds into mitochondrial oxidation via conversion to acetyl-CoA.

Aerobic Metabolism

Let's assume there is plentiful oxygen and the mitochondria are fully capable of aerobic metabolism. This changes things considerably as far as the potential to burn glucose and fat. Even though glycolysis will continue and make small amounts of energy as a sideline purpose now, the main purpose of glycolysis when mitochondria are functional is to fuel the cell. The end product, pyruvate, will not go to lactate for disposal but will go to the mitochondria, where *pyruvate dehydrogenase* will convert it to acetyl-CoA. Now we are talking energy production! The two acetyl-CoAs produced from a single glucose in glycolysis (Figure 14.1) will now go through the same TCA cycle I described in Chapter 9, on fatty acid oxidation. Through the TCA cycle—which is really the final common pathway of oxidation of glucose, fatty acids, and other metabolites—the acetyl-CoA will be oxidized, producing four NADH molecules per acetyl-CoA. Recall that in glycolysis only two molecules of NADH+H$^+$ were generated for each oxidized glucose molecule, and without oxygen they were at a dead end. Now, the output includes a further three NADH+H$^+$s and one $FADH_2$ per acetyl-CoA, or double each per-glucose equivalent, simply by using aerobic metabolism available in the mitochondria. Since oxygen is available and the mitochondria are fully functional, the mitochondria will also be carrying out an additional essential pathway of energy production: the process called oxidative-phosphorylation. Oxidative-phosphorylation now takes the $NADH+H^+$s, as well as the $ETF-FADH_2$ molecules produced from fatty acid oxidation (Chapter 9, Figure 9.3), and converts their energy into the final production of ATP. From each $NADH+H^+$ essentially three ATPs are produced, and from each $FADH_2$, two ATPs are generated. Therefore, from a single glucose going only through glycolysis the net output is two ATPs, but a single glucose going through glycolysis plus mitochondrial oxidation produces 38 high-energy phosphate molecules like ATP. Since glycolysis uses no oxygen, it is called anaerobic metabolism, and since mitochondrial oxidation uses oxygen, it is called aerobic metabolism. Realize that mitochondrial fatty acid oxidation is also part of this aerobic oxidation. Like glycolysis, if acetyl-CoAs and $NADH+H^+$s get too high because of deficient oxygen, fatty acid oxidation also stops. What a difference oxygen makes!

Oxidation and Exercise

Oxidation is the key to maintaining blood lipid concentrations and glucose concentrations in the normal range over the long haul. Insulin resistance and eventually diabetes develop over decades of rising blood glucose concentrations and increasingly elevated fatty acids and triglycerides. Remember also that the mechanisms of obesity are simple; if energy expenditure is less than energy intake, the net energy balance is displayed as excess fat. For someone who wants to reverse a state of "energy balance excess" (fatness), there are three options: (1) eat less, (2) exercise more, or (3) do both (probably the best option). Granted, genetics may have a strong influence on how easy or difficult it will be to eat less *or* exercise more. The bottom line, despite all the qualifiers, is that any calorie taken in as food must either be oxidized or stored.

Why not take a pill that revs up metabolism and simply burn off the excess fat? For one thing, your body temperature may go dangerously high! The energy a body produces must either be used for energy expenditure, like exercise, or for body heat generation. Body fat does not simply and quietly disappear, as the purveyors of so many "quack" weight-loss products suggest. In order to burn fat without any exercise, the body would have to generate body heat. This could be deadly.

Instead of a pill, therefore, our bodies rely on the natural processes of metabolism and movement to burn energy. It all started with the "flight or fight" response of epinephrine release, which triggers release of glucose from glycogen stores in the liver or in muscle cells themselves. Aerobic or oxidative metabolism yields many more ATPs than anaerobic metabolism. If the body is "yielding" ATPs in a healthy way—i.e., not drug induced—there will be a potential reduction of fat storage. A sprinter needs only the quick spurt of energy provided by glycolysis and trains for meeting this need by adapting his or her muscles to glycolytic metabolism, while the marathon runner needs full glucose and fatty acid oxidation for energy that is not necessarily needed quickly as much as it is needed over a long time period. These different runners, with different energy needs, train their muscle metabolic pathways through exercise training to be primed for their particular needs. A sprinter over time will tend to develop more white muscle (primed for glycolytic metabolism) whereas a long-distance runner will tend to have a higher proportion of red muscle to accommodate the need for oxidative metabolism.

Genetics could influence one's athletic ability and endurance. Suppose an individual with the alleles for the genes that promote for a larger proportion of white muscle versus red muscle wants to be a marathon runner. This person may be greatly frustrated unless he or she learns that sprinting is a better option. Athletes can train to increase their oxidative metabolism, but there are likely several genes that influence their makeup as well.

Increasing Resting Energy Expenditure

Some individuals may be more resistant to increased body fat gain because they have relatively higher resting energy expenditure (REE), also called resting metabolic rate (RMR). The REE is the amount of energy our bodies expend at a background burn rate. It accounts for over half or more of our daily energy expenditure (Kearney 2003). Energy expenditure from exercise is a fraction of the daily total (Speakman and Selman 2003). Thus the less exercise we do, the more important is the REE component for overall bodyweight. That is, body mass—represented by organs, fat, and muscle—burns energy at this background level. Someone who loses weight, including fat mass, will have a lower REE after the weight loss. Body organs such as brain, liver, and kidneys have higher REE than muscle or adipose tissues. The relative scale of

REE is approximately: organs (1,000–1,500 kJ/kg per day), skeletal muscle (60–125 kJ/kg per day), and adipose tissue (10–30 kJ/kg per day) (Hallgren et al. 1989; Nelson et al. 1992). Unfortunately, there is no healthy way to increase organ mass (can't "pump up" the liver) to take advantage of this.

There has been interest in attempting to increase REE through different types of exercise. One form of exercise tested was aerobic training, such as distance running. Numerous studies have investigated this approach to increasing REE with varying results. The consensus by many is that, for the average person, aerobic training will not increase REE enough to have a practical effect on body fat mass. The amount of training required is intolerable to the average person (Kearney 2003). Another type of exercise with possible effects on REE is resistance training, such as weight-lifting. Studies of resistance training have had more positive results than those reported for aerobic training (Kearney 2003). Increasing fat free mass (FFM)—namely, muscle mass—has been shown to increase REE, though REE per pound of muscle mass may not change much. The mechanism for these responses is not clear. Theoretically, adding resistance training to maintain or increase FFM (muscle) in order to maintain or increase REE should make weight loss in treatment of obesity easier to achieve and maintain. Unfortunately, however, applications of resistance training for weight loss among the obese have not been very successful (Kearney 2003).

One problem with restricting dietary calories too much, along with trying too vigorously to exercise away extra fat pounds, is that the body will resist after a while. In fact, the body may respond to an energy-demanding challenge (drastically decreasing calorie intake combined with rigorous exercise) not by burning fat but by breaking down muscle for energy maintenance. (Remember, our genotypes are designed to protect the body's fat stores.) This makes fat even harder to get rid of, despite all of the hard work and sacrifice. Using muscle-building anaerobic exercises to supplement an all-out aerobic attack on the fat may counteract this fat-burning restriction. Over time, as muscle mass and perhaps REE increases, there may be an increase in the burning of calories during resting metabolism.

Beyond body fat control, resistance training has other benefits to be considered. As we age, we tend to lose muscle, a process known as muscle atrophy or sarcopenia (Hunter, McCarthy, and Bamman 2004). Along with sarcopenia comes loss of strength. This becomes a significant problem in the elderly because of the increased risk of falls, fatigability, and difficultly with mobility. Numerous studies have indicated that older muscles adapt vigorously to resistance training with marked muscle cell hypertrophy, the opposite of sarcopenia (Hunter, McCarthy, and Bamman 2004). Another benefit of increased activity in the elderly, including resistance training, is improved bone health.

Exercise, Obesity, and Insulin Resistance

Exercise, working through the mechanisms described above, has direct relevance for what is happening in obese and insulin-resistant individuals. David Kelley, Bret Goodpaster, and colleagues have reported important studies elucidating these relationships (Goodpaster, Watkins, and Kelley 2001; Goodpaster, Katsiaras, and Kelley 2003; He, Goodpaster and Kelley 2004; Kelley 2004; Pruchnic et al. 2004). Obese, insulin-resistant individuals have excessive lipids in muscle cells (intramyocellular lipid, IMCL), with all fiber types affected. In lean individuals, muscle metabolism during a fast is characterized by a predominance of fatty acid oxidation over glucose oxidation. When lean individuals have an increase in insulin, they switch to glucose oxidation with a concomitant reduction in fatty acid oxidation. Obese individuals at baseline have abnormally low fatty acid oxidative capacity during fasting, and when they experience increased insulin concentrations in the blood they show little to no response with a change in oxidative metabolism. Sedentary obese individuals also have smaller mitochondria in muscle cells, along with a reduced capacity for fat or glucose oxidation—all of which correlates with increased insulin resistance. Basically, these individuals have little to no metabolic flexibility in comparison with lean individuals. Exercise combined with weight loss enhances fatty acid oxidation and increased insulin sensitivity in obese individuals (Goodpaster, Katsiaras, and Kelley 2003). It has been shown by many investigators that insulin-resistant individuals have an elevated accumulation of IMCL. The surprising results provided by Kelley and Goodpaster were that trained athletes also showed increased IMCL but have very good insulin sensitivity (Goodpaster, Watkins, and Kelley 2001). Thus, the IMCL probably has no direct effect on oxidative capacity; rather, it is an indicator that acyl-CoA molecules are excessive in insulin resistance. An excess of acyl-CoA may be the real culprit in development of insulin resistance, whereas in trained athletes, the acyl-CoA concentrations remain low because the molecules are oxidized—in other words, acyl-CoA remains low despite the appearance of IMCL. Obese individuals who experience weight loss along with increased fitness retain IMCL, but their basal fatty acid oxidation capacity increases along with their insulin sensitivity (He, Goodpaster, and Kelley 2004). In contrast, obese sedentary individuals who lost weight with no increased physical activity (for example, by bariatric surgery) showed decreased levels of IMCL in muscle but had no improvement in oxidative capacity for burning fat (Kelley 2004). Likewise, elderly individuals who were previously sedentary but who experienced twelve weeks of exercise training increased their IMCL as well as their oxidative capacity (Pruchnic et al. 2004). The improvement was reflected in an increased whole-body (systemic) aerobic oxidative capacity. These individuals also increased their type I muscle fibers.

Exercise, Hyperlipidemia, Metabolic Syndrome, and Cardiovascular Disease

Claude Bouchard and colleagues have carried out a major family study, called HERITAGE, designed to investigate the contribution of regular exercise to changes in the risk factors for cardiovascular disease and type 2 diabetes and also the role of genetics in the cardiovascular, metabolic, and endocrine responses to exercise training (Leon et al. 2002; Katzmarzyk et al. 2003). The study investigating HDL cholesterol changes with exercise included 675 sedentary healthy people, both black and white, both men and women, aged 17–65 years of age. These participants performed 20 weeks of supervised cycle ergometer exercise. This exercise program initially included three 30-minute sessions per week and progressed to 50-minute sessions during the final six weeks. The mean HDL values for the whole group significantly increased by 3.6%, but there was marked variability in responsiveness to exercise training. No significant differences were observed in the HDL response across sex, racial ancestry, age, or level of fitness (Leon et al. 2002). In another study, 621 black and white participants of the HERITAGE Family Study were evaluated for the diagnosis of metabolic syndrome (see Chapter 5) before undertaking the exercise training program (Katzmarzyk et al. 2003). From the group of 621 apparently healthy participants, 105 were diagnosed with metabolic syndrome. After the exercise training program, 32 (30.5%) of the original 105 no longer had signs of metabolic syndrome. Of the 32 participants who improved their metabolic profiles, 43% had decreased blood triglyceride concentrations, 16% had improved blood HDL concentrations, 38% had decreased blood pressure, 9% improved fasting blood glucose concentrations, and 28% had reduced waist circumference. There were no sex or ancestry differences in these improved metabolic profiles in response to exercise training.

In a different study, DNASCO (DNA Polymorphism and Carotid Atherosclerosis), by Bouchard and colleagues, a 6-year randomized, controlled trial of middle-aged men, investigated the effect of regular long-term physical exercise on chronic low-grade inflammation and the progression of atherosclerosis (Rauramaa et al. 2004). Aerobic exercise did not slow the progression of atherosclerosis in the participants overall, but there was significant improvement in those not taking HMG-CoA reductase inhibitors (statins) (Rauramaa et al. 2004). Statins, powerful drugs used to reduce blood cholesterol concentrations, will be discussed in the next chapter. Overall, we can take away several important points from these studies. There were several benefits of exercise for many of the participants of these large studies. Not all participants, however, demonstrated benefits for all metabolic measures evaluated. There also appeared to be the same benefits regardless of ancestry or sex, but none of the studies showed a 100% positive response in the participants.

All activity, especially exercise, uses stored energy such as glycogen and fat for fuel. Glycogen is first broken down into its component part, glucose. Glucose then goes through the anaerobic process of glycolysis, which does not make much energy. Lactic acid may build up if oxidative metabolism is not possible, and this may be experienced as "cramps." Glycogen in the liver is broken down to supply glucose to the whole body, whereas glycogen in muscle is strictly used by the muscle cell of origin. If oxygen is in good supply, and the muscle cell has sufficient mitochondria and myoglobin to transfer the oxygen supplied to it from the red blood cell's hemoglobin, this muscle cell can fully oxidize the products of glycolysis and produce the ATPs needed for vigorous muscle contraction. Likewise, muscle cells can use fatty acids, via mitochondrial oxidation, to produce large and sustained amounts of ATP. In sum, quick energy is supplied by glycolysis, and sustained energy is supplied by the breakdown of glucose and fatty acids through mitochondrial oxidative metabolism. The benefits of exercise extend beyond the depletion of stored fat to include improvements in blood lipid concentrations and insulin sensitivity. There are, for example, advantages of increased activity levels in the elderly, such as preserving muscle strength and maintaining a normal oxidative capacity, especially in the muscles. When dietary changes and exercise programs are not sufficient to address an individual's health problems, however, we turn to drugs for help, as I will discuss in the next chapter.

CHAPTER 15

Lipid-Lowering Drugs

We are constantly bombarded by advertisements for prescription and nonprescription drugs that are claimed to cure whatever ails us, but the ads rarely tell us how they work. In this chapter I describe how the common lipid-lowering drugs work to treat hypercholesterolemia, hypertriglyceridemia, and insulin resistance. The principles by which these drugs work are explained in terms of lipid metabolism. I also bring up other important issues, such as use of drugs in combination with other preventive measures—life-style changes, for example—and the common problem of patients not taking their prescribed drugs.

Prescription Drugs: A Preamble

Throughout this book I have alluded to drugs that are commonly used to treat the various maladies of excess fat. The discussions of these drugs that follow is meant to be generic, without reference to or endorsement of any particular brand of drug. It is intended entirely for providing background information about drug mechanisms and not as a recommendation for therapy.

Since 1997, the U.S. Food and Drug Administration (FDA) has regulated direct-to-consumer advertising of prescription drugs, and since then the airwaves and pages of magazines have been filled with ads urging men and women to "talk to your doctor" about this or that drug (General Accounting Office 2002). Many of these medicines are aimed at controlling blood lipid levels. My goal in this chapter is to help you understand how these drugs work

177

in terms of the different aspects of lipid metabolism and associated diseases that have been explored throughout this book.

For most of the history of the human pharmacopoeia, obesity, insulin resistance, type 2 diabetes, hyperlipidemia, and atherosclerosis were not common problems. As late as 1900, the life expectancy of an American white male was just 46.6 years. People were much more likely to die of acute illness or trauma than of chronic disease—they were carried off by cholera or diphtheria, the complications of childbirth, or a farm or factory accident before they had a chance to develop atherosclerosis. Obesity was the rare problem of the privileged few throughout history. Henry VIII, for example, purportedly had a 54-inch waist. President Theodore Roosevelt was a large man who may have had metabolic syndrome (Junod 2003). Most notorious in U.S. political history was Roosevelt's successor, President William Howard Taft, who got stuck in the White House bathtub—and later had an enormous one installed. He was close to six feet tall and weighed, at his heaviest, 340 pounds (BMI > 42); he suffered from sleep apnea, severe daytime somnolence, and hypertension (Sotos 2003). Fortunately, after leaving the presidency he lost weight and stayed at around 264 pounds the rest of his life. Although still obese, his sleep and blood pressure improved with the weight loss.

Pharmacologic approaches to treatment of diseases of excess fat have been relatively recent. In contrast to the wide array of drugs available to treat hypertension, development of anti-obesity drugs lags decades behind. This is partly because the pathophysiology of obesity and related disorders has only recently begun to be more fully understood. There is concern by many investigators that the development and clinical use of new drugs for these medical problems is too slow because of the complex regulatory pathway required to get new drugs safely on the market. There are further concerns about conflicts of interest between the investigators performing the large clinical trials and the drug companies that are paying for the trials. All of these issues are under intense public and governmental scrutiny and have a marked effect on the introduction of useful drugs.

During the past decade, clinical trials of prescription drugs have included both men and women of multiple races. This is an important improvement over drug data determined predominantly from white males, as was the practice years ago. A remaining gap in clinical drug trials is the lack of data for children and teenagers. This is becoming especially important for many of the drugs discussed in this chapter because of the high prevalence in children and teens of what used to be "adult" diseases, such as type 2 diabetes, as well as the rare but severe hereditary conditions, such as familial hypercholesterolemia (Rodenburg et al. 2004). Most pediatricians make their best estimate on "off-label" use of a medication, adjust the dose on a surface-area basis (comparing child and adult size), prescribe it, and monitor safety and efficacy.

The practice of American medicine has become very dependent on prescribing drugs while, as some would say, ignoring other avenues of disease prevention. Many are finding, however, that positive lifestyle changes accompanied by judicious use of drugs may be the most effective approach to both prevention and treatment when a disease does arise. I think American medicine has become overly dependent on expecting a pill to cure what often is a complex problem of behavior, diet, environment, and genetics. My preference is that both healthcare providers and patients rely first on preventive medicine (control weight before obesity develops, start an exercise program to avoid a problem like insulin resistance), then, if necessary, use diet and behavior modifications to reverse disease processes already under way, and only use drugs as needed.

Statins for Lowering Cholesterol

During the 1970s and 1980s, as the molecular mechanisms underlying cholesterol metabolism began to be much more fully understood, a class of drugs emerged that have proven invaluable for controlling elevated blood cholesterol concentrations, especially those due to excess LDL cholesterol (Witztum 1996; Gotto 1999; Hunninghake and Stein 2000). I mentioned earlier (Chapter 4) the important research contributions of Konrad Bloch, Feodor Lynen, John Cornforth, G. Popjak, and Robert Woodward to our understanding of cholesterol synthesis. In addition, later work by Akira Endo specifically on statins was crucial for the development of the new drugs for treatment of hypercholesterolemia (Bloch 1965; Endo 1992). Statins are officially known as 3-hydroxy-3-metylglutaryl-CoA (HMG-CoA) reductase inhibitors. The original compound, isolated from *Penicillium* species of fungus, was known as compactin; later named mevastatin, it was the first statin described, in 1976 (Endo 1992).

Several drugs from several companies fall into the "statin" category, and you have probably heard of many of them (see Table 15.1). Statins lower cholesterol levels by inhibiting the synthesis of cholesterol. Acetyl-CoAs are converted into cholesterol via a multi-step process (see Figure 4.1). Recall that the level and activity of cholesterol synthesis enzymes are extremely sensitive to the intracellular concentration of sterols or cholesterol-like molecules. As a result, when sterols are high, the cell shuts down synthesis of cholesterol and also "retracts" its LDL receptors to prevent further uptake of even more cholesterol from the blood. Statins directly affect this mechanism to lower LDL cholesterol (Figure 15.1).

Normally, if the cell has been "bathed" in excess cholesterol, and it has already imported all that it needs, it reduces LDL receptor number—as though it were thinking, "Enough cholesterol already." The first action of a statin is exactly what the name implies; it inhibits HMG-CoA reductase, the enzyme needed for the rate-limiting step of cholesterol synthesis. HMG-CoA reductase is inhibited, reducing the amount of cholesterol synthesized from that point on, and the cell "feels" cholesterol deprived. In fact, the cell is sensing the low sterol level via the SREBP mechanism, discussed earlier, and the cell's reaction is to increase the level of LDL receptors. Since the LDL receptors available on the cell surface increase in number, there is a strong pull of LDL cholesterol from the blood for disposal by the liver. The actual amount of HMG-CoA reductase is increased via the same gene expression mechanism that increases the number of LDL receptors. Although there is more enzyme present, it is inhibited by the statin (Figure 15.1). The newer, more potent statins, for example rosuvastatin, also decrease hepatic synthesis of VLDL particles, thus decreasing both VLDL and LDL particles in the blood. The combined effect would include lower LDL cholesterol as well as triglyceride concentrations in the blood. Unfortunately, we do not have the same level of detail on the mechanisms of action of most of the other drugs used in medicine.

Statins are quite remarkable: they can lower blood cholesterol concentrations, predominantly LDL cholesterol, by 20–60% in some patients (Witztum

Table 15.1. HMG-CoA reductase inhibitors ("statins")

Generic Name	Brand name	Company
Atorvastatin	Lipitor	Pfizer
Cerivastatin	Baychol[a]	Bayer
Fluvastatin	Lescol	Sandoz
Lovastatin	Mevacor	Merck
Pravastatin	Pravacol	Bristol-Meyers Squibb
Rosuvastatin	Crestor	AstraZeneca
Simvastatin	Zocor	Merck

a. Voluntarily taken off the market by Bayer (August 2001) because rhabdomyolysis, a severe reaction by the muscle, occurred in some patients.

1996; Gotto 1999; Hunninghake and Stein 2000). Lowering dietary sugars and starches, cholesterol, and saturated and *trans* fat will supplement this process, but dietary changes alone are not nearly as effective as the use of statins. As you can see from Figure 15.1, functional LDL receptors are required for statins to work maximally. So this drug is of limited to no benefit in patients who are homozygous for familial hypercholesterolemia. It sometimes helps heterozygous patients, however, if they can generate a statin-induced increased synthesis of LDL receptors from their single, fully functional LDL receptor gene.

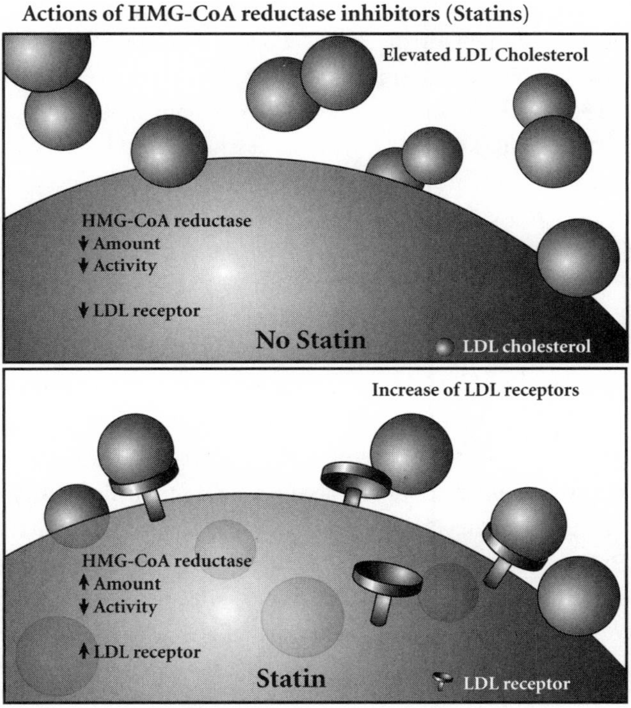

Actions of HMG-CoA reductase inhibitors (Statins)

Figure 15.1. Actions of statins and cellular cholesterol flux. The cell in the upper panel is surrounded by a high concentration of LDL cholesterol. It detects that there is plenty of cholesterol present, so it has reduced its capacity for both internal synthesis and uptake of LDL cholesterol from the outside by reducing the number of LDL receptors on its surface. The cell in the lower panel has been tricked by a statin into sensing it has little cholesterol and needs more, so the cell increases synthesizing activity by increasing the amount of HMG-CoA reductase (although this is directly inhibited by the statin). The cell also increases the number of LDL receptors in the cell membrane to reduce the LDL cholesterol outside the cell by increasing uptake into the cell.

Bile Acid Resins and Cholesterol Absorption Blockers

Beyond statins, there are some other drug tricks that can be played to lower a person's blood cholesterol. The next one is an "outside" attack, so to speak. Cholesterol exits the body via the liver in the form of bile acids. Bile acids are normally collected in the gall bladder and secreted as bile in response to food coming into the stomach and upper small intestine. The only problem with that mechanism is that more than 97% of the bile acids secreted by the liver are reabsorbed by the intestine (see Chapter 4). What if bile acids, this disposal form of cholesterol produced by the liver, remained trapped in the intestine and were sent out with the stool? This is what bile acid sequestrants, also known as "resins," do. Resins, used since the 1980s, are taken by mouth (Witztum 1996; Gotto 1999; Hunninghake and Stein 2000). They are then present in the food digesting in the small intestine, where bile is secreted, and they bind the bile acids so they cannot be recycled. This induced loss of bile acids will require more conversion of cholesterol to bile acids, so an increased number of LDL receptors are produced for the membranes of liver cells, and HMG-CoA reductase activity is stepped up as well. The liver "thinks" it is cholesterol deficient. This compensatory increase in intracellular cholesterol partly negates the benefit of preventing cholesterol from being reabsorbed, but bile acid resin alone can lower *total* cholesterol concentrations in blood by 10–20%; LDL cholesterol may decrease by 10–35%. This process sets up a net flux of cholesterol out of the body. Since the starting problem was excess cholesterol, we have no need to worry about a cholesterol deficiency. The two main bile acid resins are cholestyramine and cholestopol (Witztum 1996; Gotto 1999; Hunninghake and Stein 2000). One of the common problems with sequestrant drugs is that they can induce a feeling of being bloated and promote constipation or excess gas because of the way they work. Another problem is that their intake must be timed so as not to interfere with other drugs.

A newer drug— colesevelam (Welchol), which comes in capsules—works by a similar mechanism, but it reportedly is less likely than resins to cause constipation. Both resins and colesevelam may cause increased blood triglyceride concentrations in some patients. Given their mechanisms of action, the bile acid sequestrants are useful in FH patients, whereas statins may have little to no effect, especially in homozygous individuals. By trapping the bile acids in the intestine for removal in the stool, resins reduce the body burden of cholesterol, despite the problem that the FH patient still lacks LDL receptors. In non-FH patients, the resins can be combined very effectively with the statins for enhanced cholesterol lowering.

Another class of cholesterol-lowering drugs that block intestinal absorption includes two margarine-based compounds containing plant-derived stanols and sterols. One example of a stanol-containing product is Benecol, which reduces intestinal absorption of dietary cholesterol, not bile acids. The drug has basically the same net effect, however, the lowering of blood cholesterol. This compound comes in the form of margarine and soft gel capsules for easy intake. Ironically, Benecol margarine contains up to 0.5 gram of *trans* fat per fourteen-gram serving, despite the consumer information that says it has no *trans* fat (Benecol). As a side note, Benecol's active ingredient, sitostanol-ester, is a good example of a plant-derived compound that has been clinically tested, published in the *New England Journal of Medicine,* and marketed in a consistent preparation (Miettinen et al. 1995). It is an example in stark contrast to the concoctions I will mention in Chapter 18. The second, somewhat similar product is Take Control, a margarine containing 1.7 grams of soybean-derived sterol esters per tablespoon serving. This compound has purportedly been shown to reduce LDL cholesterol by 17% when used as directed (Take Control 2005).

In Table 15.2, I have summarized the generic names and brand names of the most commonly used drugs for lowering lipids. A very recent addition to cholesterol-lowering drugs is ezetimibe, more commonly known as Zetia. This drug selectively blocks absorption of cholesterol from the intestine. It is often used in combination with a low-dose statin to provide a marked lowering of blood cholesterol concentrations, without causing constipation as the bile acid resins do. Recently, ezetimibe has been combined with the statin simvastatin in a product called Vytorin.

Fat Blockers

There is such a thing as a fat blocker: Orlistat. The intention of prescribing this drug is not to allow patients to eat all they want and still lose weight. This drug is intended for obesity management—including weight loss and weight maintenance, in conjunction with a reduced-calorie diet—as well as reducing the risk of weight regain after loss. It is a prescription drug used mostly in extreme cases of obesity because of its cost and potential side effects. The patient characteristics include a BMI over 30 or a BMI over 27 with additional risk factors such as hypertension, diabetes, and dyslipidemia. Orlistat reportedly blocks fat absorption by approximately 30% by reversible inhibition of lipases (enzymes that "cut up" lipid molecules into smaller molecules) in the stomach and the small intestine. Patients who use this drug may experience oily diarrhea, because it traps so much fat in the stool. Unfortunately, drugs like Orlistat and other antiobesity drugs are not approved for indefinite use. That is, once an individual loses the excess weight, he or she no longer fits the criteria to be treated with the drug. Such a person would have to fatten up in order to be eligible again. There are no obesity-prevention drugs.

Niacin for Lowering Cholesterol

The next drug to discuss is probably known to you already as a B vitamin, nicotinic acid, or niacin. Nicotinic acid has been recognized as a hypolipidemic agent and used since the mid-1950s (Witztum 1996; Gotto 1999; Hunninghake and Stein 2000). As a vitamin, it is important in the formation of the enzymatic co-factors NADH and NADPH, among other functions. Recall that fatty acid oxidation, during the 3-hydroxyacyl-CoA dehydrogenase steps, requires NADH (see Figure 9.3). The effects of nicotinic acid for lowering lipids is entirely what doctors call a "pharmacologic effect," meaning that a molecu-

Table 15.2. Lipid drugs: bile acid sequestrant (resins), fibrates, and "glitazones"

Type of drug	Generic name	Brand name	Company
Bile acid sequestrants	Cholestryramine	Questran	Bristol-Meyers Squibb
	Colesevelam	Welchol	GelTex
	Cholestopol	Colestid	Pharmacia & Upjohn
Cholesterol absorption blockers	Sitostanol-ester	Benecol	McNeil Consumer Healthcare
	Ezetimibe	Zetia	Merck/Schering-Plough
Fat absorption blocker	Orlistat	Xenical	Roche
Nicotinic acid (niacin)	Nicotinic acid	Many	Many
Fibrates	Gemfibrozil	Lopid	Warner-Lambert
	Fenofibrate	Tricor	Abbott
	Clofibrate	Atromid-S	Wyeth-Ayerest
Thiazolidinediones ("glitazones")	Troglitazone[a]	Rezulin	Parke-Davis (Pfizer)
	Pioglitazone	Actos	Takeda/Eli Lilly
	Rosiglitazone	Avandia	GlaxoSmithKline
Other insulin sensitizers	Metformin	Glucaphage	Bristol-Myers Squibb

a. Voluntarily taken off the U.S. market by Parke-Davis division of Warner Lambert on March 21, 2000, because of liver failure in a small number of patients.

lar compound, or drug, is used in high doses to get a desired effect, and these effects often have nothing to do with the normal function of the compound when it is taken in the usual amount. In the case of using nicotinic acid for lowering lipids, the mechanism of action is mostly unknown. Researchers think its action is caused in part by the ability of nicotinic acid to reduce lipolysis, which leads to a net reduction of the blood concentrations of free fatty acids that would normally go to the liver and be repackaged as VLDLs. The overall output by the liver of VLDLs is lowered, and therefore VLDL remnants and LDLs are also decreased. Nicotinic acid may also increase the lipoprotein lipase activity, since it is the enzyme that cleaves the fatty acids free from triglycerides found in the VLDL particles. Thus, the net effect is to reduce VLDL synthesis, because there is an overall lower level of triglyceride building up in the liver to be exported, and to increase clearance of the VLDL triglycerides.

Nicotinic acid has many positive features. It is relatively cheap to take, and in many people it can increase HDL levels while decreasing LDL and VLDL concentrations. Nicotinic acid is one of the most effective ways to raise blood HDL concentrations. There are down sides to consider, though. A person has to take 2–6 grams per day, which is a lot to swallow. For example, a standard ibuprofen tablet delivering 200 milligrams of active ingredient weighs 0.324 grams. A six-gram dose of nicotinic acid would equal the mass of 18.5 ibuprofen tablets. One other down side is that 50% of patients who take these large doses of nicotinic acid have side effects of flushing and itching of the skin. Fortunately, after a while the itching and flushing subside in many patients, yet the benefits of this high dose of nicotinic acid continue. Another major side effect is liver toxicity; patients must be monitored while taking the drug. Some slow-release forms of nicotinic acid are most prone to this effect (Henkin, Johnson, and Segrest 1990). The mechanism of toxicity remains unknown, but it may be related to the more extended blood level obtained or the differences in the sites of intestinal absorption of the nicotinic acid.

Fibrates for Lowering Blood Triglycerides

Another group of lipid-lowering drugs is the fibrates (Witztum 1996; Gotto 1999; Hunninghake and Stein 2000). Fibrates are often used for lowering abnormally high blood triglycerides. They were originally studied in rats and found to be potent lipid-lowering agents in the early 1960s (Witztum 1996). When given fibrates in large doses, the rats developed liver enlargement and low blood lipids (hypolipidemia). Their livers enlarged because of a proliferation of a small cellular organelle known as the peroxisome. (Fibrates eventually became known as peroxisomal proliferators.) Although the functions of the peroxisome remain a bit of an enigma, some of its known functions include β-oxidation of very long-chain fatty acids (with more than 20 carbons) and synthesis of bile acids and specialized lipids crucial for the nervous system.

It was later discovered that peroxisomal proliferators (PPs) increased peroxisome numbers and lowered blood lipids via a protein named the peroxisomal proliferator–activated receptor (PPAR). The main PPAR in the liver is PPAR-α, and it is the one that responds to fibrate drugs and fatty acids (Schoonjans, Staels, and Auwerx 1996). The overall effect of PPAR-α activation by a fibrate is threefold: (1) increased fatty acid uptake and oxidation via peroxisomes and mitochondria (see Figure 9.3); (2) decreased expression of apolipoprotein C-III and lowered incorporation of this lipoprotein derivative into VLDL, which results in increased lipoprotein lipase activity to clear blood triglycerides from VLDL; and (3) decreased overall VLDL synthesis by the liver due to more burning of fatty acids, therefore leaving fewer available to form triglycerides and also lowering blood triglycerides. Although the fibrates are often used to reduce blood triglycerides, they also have other effects on the blood concentrations of cholesterol-carrying lipoproteins. In many patients fibrates may increase or decrease LDL cholesterol and may increase HDL concentrations slightly.

Shown in Figure 15.2 is an overview of the desired effects of proper PPAR functioning and the ways fibrates can induce these effects. The two drug classes illustrated here appear to be activating pathways that normally should be activated by fatty acids. Further study has shown that these actions are best promoted by long-chain omega-3 fatty acids (fish oil fatty acids, as described back in Chapter 2). These two drugs seem to be activating a pathway that could be stimulated by dietary fatty acids such as fish oil. Additional benefits of fish oil omega-3 fatty acids include reduction in both inflammatory processes and clotting, which mitigates the disease processes involved in atherogenesis and myocardial infarctions.

Drugs for Increasing Insulin Sensitivity

In Chapter 6 the thiazolidinediones (TZDs), otherwise known as the "glitazones," made an appearance. First used in the mid-1990s, these drugs increase insulin sensitivity by lowering blood concentrations of free fatty acids. The full range of mechanisms is not fully understood, but it looks as if a major component of the glitazone function resides in their ability to activate PPAR-γ in adipose tissue. It appears that after the glitazones activate PPAR-γ, it in turn activates a whole series of genes that promote for triglyceride storage in adipose tissue. This drug also seems to increase the number of adipocytes to store the increasing load of fatty acids. These drugs seem to work remarkably well, although the long-term effects of lowering free fatty acids in the blood at the cost of increasing adipose storage of fat remain to be seen. In recent studies of mice done by my research team, we found another possible mechanism not previously reported; at least one of the drugs, rosiglitazone, increased the expression of fatty acid oxidation genes in adipose tissue (Goetzman et al. 2003). The fat burning that results could also help dispose of excess fatty acids in the blood without adding more triglyceride to storage. Most patients who take these drugs tend to gain weight, although their blood glucose is under better control as a result of improved insulin sensitivity. Some patients gain weight because of increased adipose tissue deposition, and some gain weight because of increased fluid retention as edema if they have underlying heart disease. Judging by their mechanism of action, I consider the TZDs a lipid-lowering drug class since they appear to function by lowering free fatty acid concentrations in the blood.

Another drug commonly used in type 2 diabetes patients is called metformin, first introduced in 1957 (Zhou et al. 2001). This drug increases the pa-

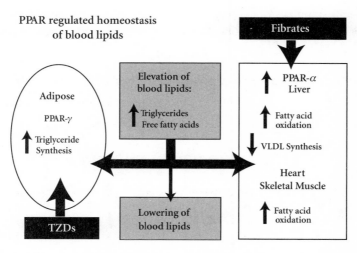

Figure 15.2. These are the desirable effects of lowering the concentration of free fatty acids in the blood. Fibrates activate PPAR-α to stimulate fatty acid oxidation in liver and muscle while the glitazones, or TZDs, activate PPAR-γ to trap fatty acids in adipose tissue.

tient's sensitivity to insulin, as do the glitazones, but through a different mechanism. Metformin appears to activate an enzyme known as AMP-activated protein kinase (AMPK) (Figure 15.3) (Zhou et al. 2001). That name tells us that this enzyme, under certain conditions, attaches a phosphate to other proteins. Attachment of a phosphate often activates or inactivates the protein. Metformin activates AMPK, which then inactivates other critical enzymes that regulate lipid and glucose metabolism. The net effect is that acetyl-CoA carboxylase is inactivated, so there is a reduction in malonyl-CoA. Recall that malonyl-CoA inhibits fatty acid oxidation, and it is also the building block for fatty acid synthesis. Taking the brakes off fatty acid oxidation helps clear the liver of excess fat. Fatty acid synthesis is inhibited further because SREBP-1, the signal that normally stimulates fatty acid synthesis, is reduced when AMPK is activated by metformin. Two other key effects include decreased glucose production by the liver and increased glucose uptake and oxidation by the muscle. Therefore, the net effect is fourfold: (1) increased fatty acid oxidation, (2) decreased fatty acid synthesis, with the resulting effects of (3) lowered blood glucose following a reduction of glucose synthesis in the liver, and (4) increased metabolism of glucose in muscle. Overall, these effects promote for increase insulin sensitivity.

Case History

An overall summary of the expected effects of the drugs discussed in this chapter is shown in Table 15.3. The final point I wish to make about drugs

Metformin mechanisms of action to increase insulin sensitivity

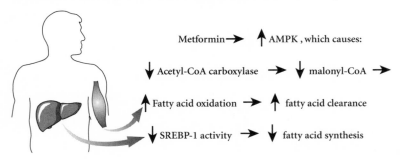

Figure 15.3. Effects of metformin on steps of metabolism that improve insulin sensitivity by decreasing fatty acids, reducing hepatic glucose output, and increasing glucose disposal.

that affect lipid metabolism is demonstrated in this case history, presented here with some details disguised.

On July 25 patient A.G., a 30-year-old white male, came to the Lipid Clinic for evaluation of his elevated blood cholesterol. Prior to the visit his blood was drawn for analysis of blood lipids. At a followup visit on October 25, he had an additional blood lipid analysis. His blood cholesterol values are shown in Table 15.4.

The patient stated that he had had high cholesterol since he was 12 years old and that his mother had died at age 48 of a heart attack. He reported that he had been taking 1 gram of niacin and 80 milligrams of simvastatin (a statin) daily. On September 9, he was further evaluated for coronary artery disease by angiography. He was diagnosed with an occluded right coronary ar-

Table 15.3. Summary of lipid and insulin sensitizer drugs and their effects on blood lipids

Drug class	Total cholesterol	LDL cholesterol	HDL cholesterol	Triglycerides
Statins	⇓⇓	⇓⇓⇓	⇑	⇓
Bile acid sequestrants	⇓	⇓⇓	⇑	NC/↑
Cholesterol absorption blockers	⇓	⇓	⇑	⇓
Nicotinic acid	⇓	⇓⇓	⇑⇑⇑	⇓⇓
Fibrates	⇓	⇓↑	⇑⇑	⇓⇓⇓
Glitazones	↑⇓	↑⇓	⇑	⇓⇓
Metformin	⇓	⇓	NC	⇓⇓

Note: These are general responses (↓ or ↑ = minor effect, ↓↓ or ↑↑ = moderate effect, ↓↓↓ or ↑↑↑ = major effect; NC = no change). The dose given of a specific drug in the class, its combination with other drugs, and individual responses may vary widely. This information represents a consensus derived from Levy, Troendle, and Fattu (1993), Witztum (1996), Gotto (1999), Lebovitz (1999), Goldberg, Semenkovich, and Ginsberg (2000), and Hunninghake and Stein (2000).

Table 15.4. Blood cholesterol values

Blood lipid (mg/dl)	July 10	October 25	Recommended values
Total cholesterol	293	134	< 200
LDL cholesterol	251	95	< 130
VLDL cholesterol	9	6	< 30
HDL cholesterol	33	37	> 40

tery. He was then prescribed 2 grams of niacin and 80 milligrams of atorvastatin (a statin). At the next blood lipid evaluation, his lipid profile had improved remarkably (Table 15.4). In fact, his results were so much better that the blood measurements were repeated for fear of a blood sample mix-up. The results were low on the second sample as well. What happened? Did simply increasing the niacin and changing to a different statin make that much difference?

The group of us who reviewed this case decided that the best explanation was that, although this patient had reported that he was taking his medicines at the earlier visit, he really was not. We speculated that perhaps, after he had had his angiography and remembered his mother dying so young, he was scared into taking his medicines. He certainly had a very positive effect from the drugs, but not necessarily because of the switch in prescriptions. The point of this case is to demonstrate that if prescribed medicines are actually taken, they can be of crucial benefit to the patient. They might even save a life.

Drugs are not always effective, but the best chance that they will be will occur if the medicine is taken as prescribed. It is estimated that anywhere from 20 to 80% of patients do not follow their doctor's treatment plan (Jaret 2001). A recent study found that only 52% of patients were still filling their prescriptions for lipid-lowering drugs after five years (Jaret 2001). Patient compliance is a major problem. So even prescribing a pill—the easiest treatment option— does not work all the time.

Alternatives to Prescription Drugs

Many people are critical of prescription drugs and prefer alternative approaches such as herbal remedies and "natural" food supplements. These treatments appear to be more "natural" because they do not seem to rely on drugs. I would caution that some of the so-called herbal and other natural food supplements are nothing more than "drugs" poorly tested both for efficacy and safety. In Chapter 18 I will return to this issue. Here I will simply offer the caveat that many alternative medicines have little to no research backing them up, and they may not work.

This chapter has introduced the drugs commonly used to treat lipid disorders. These include the statins, bile acid resins, and nicotinic acid for elevated blood cholesterol, primarily for elevated LDL cholesterol. Fibrates reduce high blood triglycerides via the PPAR-α mechanism that results in increased "burning" of fatty acids and reduced synthesis and circulation time of triglyceride-containing VLDL particles. Glitazones increase insulin sensitivity by reducing blood concentrations of free fatty acids by promoting for the storage of fatty acids in the adipose tissue. Another insulin-sensitizer, metformin, also acts to lower fatty acids in the tissues.

Proponents of the Human Genome Project, as well as many others, look forward to the day when all genes have been identified, including the important "obesity" and "diabetes" genes, and that new, pivotal drug targets will be developed through our knowledge of the biologic functions of these genes. Ideally, individualized medicine will someday evolve so that each patient's genomic "readout" will allow physicians to prescribe a drug with confidence that it will be effective and nontoxic for that patient. Until that day arrives, we must continue to piece together what is known about how fat works in health and disease. In the next chapter, I present a view of the whole picture of lipid metabolism and its disorders.

CHAPTER 16

Practical Lessons for Making Good Decisions

Excessive fat—in adipose tissues, blood, or body organs—is a serious problem. Diseases of excess fat take a high personal toll for the patient and the family and a devastating social and economic toll. This chapter puts into perspective the many aspects of excess fat, disease development, and related health risks. Much of what I have covered in this book is summarized by what I call a "fatocentric" model of the processes involved in obesity, insulin resistance, metabolic syndrome, and diabetes. It is crucial to reverse these processes. I provide a recap of the drugs commonly used to treat these disorders when genetics, age, diet, and inactivity are difficult to overcome. Finally, I argue that fitness should be everyone's goal, not only as a remedy for obesity but also to reduce the risks of many other common and devastating diseases, such as hypertension, arthritis, and osteoporosis.

Confronting Diseases of Excess Fat

We have covered a lot of ground together in this book. My goal was to teach you about the critical influences of nutrition, genetics, exercise, and drugs on body fat characteristics. I covered the different types of lipids that make up the fats in our foods and bodies. I told you about the rare and the much too common diseases that directly involve fat metabolism. I also described studies in which the genetics of these conditions are being investigated and the benefits of knowing the genes involved. Finally, I discussed the drugs commonly used to treat the disorders of too much fat. In the next and final section of the book, I will venture into new topics, such as food labels, "miracle disease cures," and how the news media can affect our understanding of health.

We have become a nation of overweight citizens at very high risk of developing insulin resistance, metabolic syndrome, type 2 diabetes, cardiovascular disease, hypertension, and many other serious maladies. In 2003, it was estimated that 65% of the U.S. population was either overweight or obese! That is a staggering statistic. It is based on the definition in which BMI values between 18.5 and 25 are "normal," BMI values of 25.1–30 are interpreted as a sign of overweight, and a BMI greater than 30 indicates obesity. You should know, however, that some obesity researchers dispute the claim that America is experiencing an epidemic of obesity (Friedman 2003).

Epidemic or not, diseases of excess fat are serious business. There are many explanations as to how the increase in these diseases has occurred, and who is to blame, and some interesting books tackle those subjects (Schlosser 2001; Shell 2002; Critser 2003). Individual action can be guaranteed to fail unless we make wider social changes. Some argue that obesity is simply an issue of individual will, but it must also be recognized that we live in a highly toxic media environment. Our individual wills are not helped by the constant intrusion of advertising for unhealthy products, which we are often misled into purchasing. We all give in to convenience rather than quality. We need to focus on high-quality unprocessed food choices that combine high fiber, healthy fats, and healthy carbohydrates. I have had personal experiences discussing re-

---

How Real Is the Obesity Epidemic?

Jeffrey Friedman, whom we met in the introductory chapter as the discoverer of leptin, was quoted in the *New York Times* as saying that the obesity epidemic we hear about daily is an illusion (Kolata 2004). He argues that the average weight of the population has increased by just 7–10 pounds since 1991. He points out that persons considered massively obese are the ones that have had a substantial increase in weight—by 25–30 pounds. Marion Nestle in the same article disagrees, saying that "everyone notices that there are more overweight people now." Friedman goes on to say, "bodyweight is genetically determined, as tightly regulated as height. Genes control not only how much you eat but also the metabolic rate at which you burn food. When it comes to eating, free will is an illusion."

search with several different food companies. There are some outstanding companies that are sincerely interested in providing healthy products and products that will help people deal with the challenges of losing weight and maintaining health. Unfortunately also, in my experience, there are too many other companies that are interested in finding some trivial health benefit to a product that in my opinion is clearly a health disaster or in avoiding negative publicity about their products. A plethora of diets, pills, creams, and exercise machines are available to consumers that supposedly help cure these ills. Some work for sound reasons, and many are nothing but gimmicks.

So what would a less toxic environment look like? What kind of environment would help with these health problems related to excess fat? Government and other community organizations could help individuals by putting policies and plans into place such as: increase safe common areas for recreation, provide sidewalks and pedestrian walkways with covers for inclement weather, provide walking and bike paths, eliminate soft drink deals and vending machines in schools, reduce crime so that grocery stores remain in low-income areas, restore public funding for physical education in schools, make it easier for people to find and purchase high-quality and low-cost local produce, dairy, meat, and fish. The profit motive drives the decisions that affect many of these issues, but a stronger focus on health would go a long way toward creating safe opportunities to be more active and purchase less commercially processed food.

The main goal of this book is to help you, as a future or present healthcare provider or inquiring citizen, realize that excess fat is a serious condition. Many folk are sitting time bombs: for some, a presently silent disease will explode into a life-threatening condition; others may already be fighting serious disease daily. I also wanted to provide you with basic information about the important issues surrounding the problems of excess body fat, so you can make good choices and effectively use these fat-reducing concepts to improve health. My thesis is that the more we all collectively understand about the factors (genetics, nutrition, activity, drugs) that influence body fat characteristics and associated diseases, the better we will be at preventing, reversing, and treating these diseases, whether in patients or in ourselves.

Criteria of a Healthy Phenotype

In Table 16.1 I have provided the normal values for blood concentrations of the metabolites covered throughout these chapters. These should be considered generic: different laboratories may have slightly different normal ranges, values change over time, and some patients with different risks, like a previous heart attack or diabetes, may need to consider lower values for LDL cholesterol, as an example. Other than HDL cholesterol, the lower these values are, the better. Lower concentrations indicate lower risks for cardiovascular disease, with the exception that higher HDL cholesterol is more favorable. Any values provided by the healthcare provider should be discussed in light of the patient's complete medical condition.

Excess body fat is obviously the result of excess stored fat and not enough fat burned for energy expenditure. The overall scenario, I believe, unfolds something like this. As people age, their overall oxidative metabolism slows. This has been shown in many studies, in many different ways. Our genomes also impose certain inherited characteristics that influence many aspects of fat metabolism, such as the overall propensity for oxidative metabolism; muscle mass; how easily or with difficulty individuals synthesize, store, and burn fat; how efficiently they absorb nutrients; and so on. We can do nothing about aging and genetics.

For whatever the reasons that people eat beyond true hunger, they begin to take in more calories than they expend. The general western diet likely contains calories predominantly from fats (excessive saturated and *trans* fats) and readily available carbohydrates, such as sugars, high-fructose corn syrup, and starch. Insulin is secreted in response to glucose derived from the carbohydrates. Interestingly, fructose does not elicit an insulin response; from the point of view of the pancreatic β-cells, fructose is a stealth sugar. Insulin stimulates the direct storage of dietary fat and the synthesis of more fat from carbohydrate sources and inhibits fat burning. Thus, insulin puts the body in energy-storage mode. If insulin is secreted repeatedly throughout the day, day in and day out, fat begins to add up. So far the body is responding as designed, but the net effect is the development of obesity. Depending on where the fat first builds up, in the butt or in the gut, many people get away with adding fat

Table 16.1. Desirable blood metabolite values (fasting)

Total cholesterol (VLDL, LDL, HDL, etc.)	< 200 mg/dl
LDL cholesterol	< 100 mg/dl
HDL cholesterol	> 40 mg/dl men
	> 50 mg/dl women
Triglycerides	< 150 mg/dl
Glucose	< 100 mg/dl

Note: Recommendations may vary depending on the patient's medical condition.

without having health problems for years. They may look fatter, but their body is maintaining normal blood glucose concentrations, although it may require more insulin. Recall from Chapter 1 that most but not all researchers believe there is a strong association between excess fat in the gut (visceral obesity) and development of insulin resistance. This sets the stage for developing the metabolic syndrome, previously known as syndrome X. In Figure 16.1 I have summarized the interrelationships among excessive calorie intake, obesity, and excessive fat synthesis, which may develop into a vicious circle leading to further development of insulin resistance and eventually diabetes.

Visceral fat is very responsive to signals for fat breakdown, or lipolysis. When lipolysis occurs in excess, it seems to act as a constant source of excess fatty acids entering the blood and going directly to the liver. The liver has

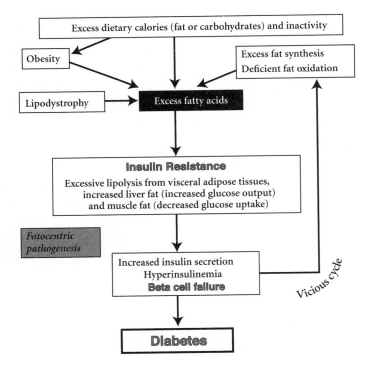

Figure 16.1. The central role of excess fatty acids in the development of insulin resistance. As insulin resistance develops, it sets in motion a vicious cycle of promoting for more insulin resistance. Exercise, reduction in calories, and drugs that lower blood fatty acids will all reverse this process.

three options on how to handle the extra fatty acids. The liver can: (1) burn fatty acids for energy production, (2) store fatty acids by converting them to triglycerides, and (3) export them as triglycerides incorporated into VLDLs. With dietary conditions characterized by frequent insulin secretion and its inhibitory effects on fat burning, fat burning is not a likely option. Metabolic syndrome, with its hallmark feature of insulin resistance, is extremely common in middle-age people, and many do not even know they have it.

I described the definitions used to diagnose metabolic syndrome back in Chapter 5. I want to repeat here that if insulin resistance can be reduced, most if not all of the other problems of metabolic syndrome will also be reversed or at least reduced.

Increase Insulin Sensitivity

Reducing the levels of fatty acids often increases insulin sensitivity. Burning these fatty acids through exercise will lower the concentration. Another way is to reduce caloric intake. Lowering caloric intake by increasing healthy fat intake seems like a paradox to many. I explained a great deal about this in Chapter 13, but let me re-emphasize several points made there. I have no argument that fat has twice the caloric density of carbohydrates, 9.3 versus 4.1 kilocalories per gram. The key point is that excess carbohydrates stimulate insulin secretion as well as appetite in many people, whereas fats do not. So by eating more healthy fats and fewer simple carbohydrates (sugars and starches), a person can control hunger while at the same time reducing calorie intake. Some healthy fats, such as the omega-3 fatty acids found in fish, may even increase fatty acid burning and reduce fatty acid synthesis. This is exactly opposite of what happens when too much insulin is secreted in response to too many carbohydrates. If some people can lower their calorie intake by eating a lot of carbohydrates, then more power to them, but for many, including yours truly, an increase in appetite overcomes any advantages of eating low-fat, high-carbohydrate foods. Any way of eating that will lower caloric intake will help these problems.

People have different sensitivities to macronutrients like fat and carbohydrates. I know of people who thought the Atkins diet was a license to gorge on steaks and sour cream, but no one will lose weight and lower their blood lipids with that approach. I have known both lean and obese vegetarians. Diets should be tools to reduce caloric intake without increasing hunger, or the diet will not work. A better concept is to find a way of eating that accomplishes one's weight-loss goals and forget about it being a "diet." Diets too often are temporary. What is really needed is a long-term lifestyle change in eating behavior. Some people may need to experiment a bit to find what reduces their hunger best. There is no one perfect diet for everyone.

There have been several randomized interventional trials, such as the Lyon Heart Study and other variations on a Mediterranean-like diet (high in whole grains, olive oil, fish, vegetables, and fruit) accompanied by lifestyle changes (increased activity), for prevention of cardiovascular disease, metabolic syndrome, or type 2 diabetes. Two recent dietary studies were carried out in an elderly population and in a group with metabolic syndrome. The study by Knoops and colleagues (2004) found that adherence to a Mediterranean diet, along with other healthy lifestyle choices, by individuals 70–90 years of age was associated with a reduction in mortality by 50% (all causes and cause-specific mortality, including coronary heart disease, cardiovascular disease, and cancer). Likewise, Esposito and colleagues (2004) compared the effect of a Mediterranean diet with that of a low-fat control diet on patients with metabolic syndrome. After two years on the diets, the patients who followed the Mediterranean diet showed greater improvement than the control group in cardiovascular disease risk factors. Some studies of the Mediterranean diet predict an associated 83% reduction in the rate of coronary heart disease, 91% reduction in diabetes in women, and 71% reduction in colon cancer in men (Rimm and Stampfer 2004). At the risk of oversimplifying, these and other studies can be summarized as follows. Perhaps a consensus view is that the healthiest diet would be high in fruit and vegetables, supplemented with fish and poultry but limited red meats, high in whole grains, high in low-fat dairy products, high in nuts, and moderate in alcohol intake. Eating this collection of different foods would provide a high percentage of monounsaturated and omega-3 long-chain fatty acids, low saturated fat, high fiber, low added sugars and starch, and low sodium. The other key factor is quantity of total calorie intake. I agree with the developing view in the nutrition field that we should focus on the entire dietary pattern rather than individual macronutrients (high this and low that) for maximum chronic disease prevention. It is clear that people are mostly unsuccessful at following a particular diet plan.

What to Do with Excess Fat

If excess fat is already present, perhaps the first thing to do about that is find a new eating pattern that works, one that reduces caloric take without increasing hunger. Losing weight, even just 5% of current weight, significantly reduces blood lipids, improves insulin sensitivity, and reduces most of the overall risks for cardiovascular disease and diabetes. I would encourage everyone to find some exercise that is enjoyable and convenient to do. Find an exercise partner for mutual support. If exercise is a dreaded ordeal, it won't last long. Endurance exercise (long jogs) burns more fat; yet resistance exercise (weightlifting) increases muscle mass, which has many advantages, as discussed earlier, especially in older individuals. Increasing muscle mass increases resting energy expenditure, which keeps more calories burning all the time; however, it takes a major increase in muscle mass to make a considerable contribution to fat loss. Thus, doing both types of exercise is optimal. Recall how few calories are actually burned during exercise. While always beneficial, exercise works better for keeping weight off once it is lost, but it is relatively inefficient at getting weight off to start with. Reduction of caloric intake is much more effective, and doing both is optimal.

Diet and exercise are sometimes not enough to achieve weight loss. In my view, the next steps are medical treatment with drugs and, if that does not work, stomach (gastric) bypass surgery. Of course, a medical treatment plan should be developed with a physician or other qualified healthcare provider. As mentioned in Chapter 15, among the options are drugs that help reduce cholesterol (statins, bile acid resins, and absorption blockers); reduce triglyceride (fibrates); increase insulin sensitivity (glitazones, metformin); and reduce fat absorption (orlistat). Gastric bypass surgery, the most drastic but a highly effective solution, is reserved only for the morbidly obese patient (BMI > 35) who has other disease risk factors, such as diabetes. This surgery markedly reduces the stomach size, which forces a drastic reduction in food intake by making it extremely uncomfortable to overeat. The result is major weight loss and a lowering of insulin resistance and high blood triglycerides within days. One problem that sometimes occurs in these patients is that losing too much body fat too fast puts extreme pressure on the liver to handle the large amount of incoming fat. Bypass surgery is a drastic measure for life-threatening cases of extreme obesity.

Genetics and Fat

Genetics clearly has major influences on body fat phenotypes. The rare inherited diseases of fat and cholesterol metabolism, as well as obesity, are straightforward, single-gene deficiencies that are inherited in the Mendelian fashion. In contrast, the common forms of obesity, dyslipidemia, insulin resistance, and diabetes are not straightforward. These diseases are caused by a complex, multifactorial process of gene-gene and gene-environment interactions. By using SNP analysis in families with these diseases, geneticists are pursuing identification of the genes involved. Once the genes are elucidated, family members could be screened and tested for genetic risk of these diseases. Furthermore, understanding more completely the different steps of metabolism and their regulation as revealed by genetics will provide new targets for drugs that might be used to treat patients when diet and exercise are not successful. Geneticists also hope to find genes that determine the effectiveness and toxicity potentials of drugs.

Fit after Fifty

Age is no reason to avoid an active lifestyle. There are many lean and fit people age fifty-plus in our society. Some are lucky. They seem to eat a lot and exercise little, while still remaining lean. Most of us are not so lucky. There are others who control caloric intake to match their energy output and can maintain their body weight at a healthy level. Weight control is key to maintaining lower blood lipids and preventing or reversing insulin resistance (metabolic syndrome). Before making drastic changes, other than simply cutting back or increasing exercise intensity, a person who wants to lose weight should consult a physician. Starting the Atkins' diet or taking a 15-mile jog may not be wise for someone with an underlying disease condition. Staying fit also makes people more resistant to other age-associated changes, such as hypertension, arthritis, and osteoporosis, to mention a few.

As I said earlier, we have covered a lot of information in our journey together through the processes of fat metabolism and its associated diseases. Clearly, it gets harder as we age to maintain a lean body status, yet it is critical to do so if you want to prevent obesity, insulin resistance, metabolic syndrome, cardiovascular disease and many other disorders. Balancing caloric intake with caloric expenditure is the key.

We have now completed the basic science portion of the book. In the final section I wish to discuss a few key issues that are relevant to our understanding of nutrition, drugs, and health care. I wrote this section as a scientist-observer, rather than as a clinical investigator on the front lines of patient care. Whether you are a research scientist, a healthcare practitioner, or an interested citizen, these issues are worth thinking about.

PART IV

The Environment

CHAPTER 17

Nutrient Labeling

While almost everyone will agree that what we eat is important for weight control and health in general, few people know how to put that knowledge into practice at the grocery store. This chapter will review what goes into producing a food package label and how to use the information provided.

Food Labels

In the United States, the labeling of food packages has been regulated by the Food and Drug Administration (FDA) since 1973 (Kurtzweil 1993; Bender, Rader, and McClure 1998). The first regulations required the labeling of foods with added nutrients and of foods that made a nutrition claim on the label or in advertising. The expanded mandate for labeling virtually all foods began in 1990, under the authority of the Nutrition Labeling and Education Act (NLEA). The FDA recommends that the nutrient values printed on the labels be based on product composition, as determined by laboratory analysis of each nutrient using the Official Methods of the Association of Official Analytical Chemists International. In order to ensure these values are accurate, the FDA periodically analyzes samples randomly collected from product lots of the various packaged foods (Bender, Rader, and McClure 1998). In addition to packaged foods, under these rules, voluntary nutrition information is made available for raw foods, including the 20 most frequently eaten raw fruits, vegetables, and fish, plus the 45 best-selling cuts of meat (FDA 1999).

The first thing at the top of the label is the serving size and the number of calories per serving. According to the FDA, NLEA defines serving size as the amount of food customarily eaten at one meal, and it must be given in common household and metric units (FDA 1999). Still, beware of the serving size! That is, calorie content may look pretty good until you realize that the serving size is only a quarter or a half of what most of us would consider a regular serving. For example, who eats only a half-cup of ice cream? One half-cup is the standard serving size listed on ice cream labels. Foods, like brownies, that have little water and have a high sugar and fat content will be very calorie rich or in other words have high caloric density. Foods high in water and fiber and low in fat, such as fruits and vegetables, will have a much lower caloric density.

At the top on the food label is the fat content. The label may list total and saturated fat, sometimes mono- and polyunsaturated fats, and cholesterol. Briefly, to review the differences in those fats from Chapter 3: saturated fat is composed of fatty acids that have no double bonds, and it is commonly derived in the highest concentrations from animal sources. Also recall that hydrogenation of vegetable oils produces *trans* fatty acids, which, like saturated fatty acids, are solid at room temperature. That is why *trans* fats are used to

Nutrition Facts		
Serving Size: 1 piece (28g)		
Servings Per Container 12		
Amount per serving		
Calories 80	Fat Cal 50	
	% Daily Value*	
Total Fat 6g	9%	
Saturated Fat 3g	15%	
Cholesterol 15mg	5%	
Sodium 200mg	8%	
Total Carb. Less Than 1g	0%	
Dietary Fiber 0g	0%	
Sugars 0g	0%	
Protein 7g		
Vitamin A 4%	Vitamin C 0%	
Calcium 20%	Iron 0%	
*Percent Daily Values are based on a 2000 calorie diet. Your daily values may be higher or lower depending on your calorie needs:		
Calories:	2000	2500
Total Fat Less than	65g	80g
Sat. Fat Less than	20g	25g
Cholesterol Less than	300mg	300mg
Sodium Less than	2,400mg	2,400mg
Total Carb.	300g	375g
Dietary Fiber	25g	30g

Figure 17.1. Food label for mozzarella cheese sticks.

harden margarine and many popular brands of peanut butter. Of all the fats mentioned here, *trans* fats are probably the most harmful to health, yet at this writing they are not listed on the food label. This information will be required as of January 1, 2006. The stiff properties of *trans* fatty acids are also characteristic of cholesterol, often associated with development of cardiovascular disease. Several studies have shown that body fat often reflects characteristics of what an animal has eaten. Someone who eats a high proportion of saturated fat and cholesterol, in the long term, will quite possibly have body fat of the same stiff consistency, which may influence his or her cardiovascular health.

In 2002, Hu and Willett summarized many studies on dietary fats (Hu and Willett 2002). In general, increasing saturated fat in the diet increases total cholesterol and LDL cholesterol in the blood, while increasing polyunsaturated fats decreases both. Replacing carbohydrates with saturated, monounsaturated, or polyunsaturated fats increases HDL, with saturated fat having a slightly greater effect. Increasing *trans* fat increases LDL cholesterol and decreases HDL cholesterol—both are changes in the wrong direction.

Beware of the label advertising low-fat or no-fat foods. In many cases, extra sugar or high-fructose corn syrup has been added to make the food tasty, so even without the fat the calorie content is still high. There are some low-fat to no-fat foods that have a higher caloric density than the traditional fat-containing version! Thus, the type of fat in the diet might affect blood lipid measurements, but calorie for calorie, dietary fat may not necessarily make anyone more or less prone to obesity.

The top number for carbohydrates on nutrition labels includes both absorbable (sugars and starches) and nonabsorbable (fiber) carbohydrates. A measure that has become known as "impact carbs" can be estimated by subtracting the grams of fiber from the total carbohydrates. This in most cases is the amount of simple sugars and starches in the food, the carbohydrates that will promote for insulin secretion.

The food label tells not only how much total fiber is provided, but some labels also give the percentage of soluble fiber. The healthful properties of oats are due to the relatively high quantity of soluble fiber found in them. A one-half cup (40 grams dry mass) serving of oats contains 4 grams of total fiber, 2 grams of that being soluble fiber. Plant cell wall components such as cellulose, hemicellulose, lignin, gums, pectins, and pentosans constitute some of the common fiber components found in foods. Humans cannot digest these fibers; it is the gut bacteria that digest the fiber. Unfortunately, this action is the source of gas that develops when individuals consume large amounts of fiber. The general understanding is that total fiber helps keep bowel movements regular because the fiber retains water, and water keeps the intestinal contents moving, thus reducing the time in transit for carcinogens that may induce colon cancer.

The insoluble fibers, cellulose and lignin found in wheat bran, are most beneficial for intestinal passage of feces. The soluble fibers—such as the gums and pectin found in fruits and legumes—are considered "heart healthy" because they help reduce LDL cholesterol in the blood. It is thought that soluble fiber slows the diffusion and absorption of cholesterol, thus keeping more cholesterol in the gut. Soluble fiber also may slow stomach emptying and delay the after-eating *(postprandial)* rise in blood glucose.

Of course, it takes years of healthy eating to reap the benefits of a high-fiber diet, such as preventing cancer or cardiovascular disease. If someone is diagnosed with polyps of the colon at age 65, it likely will not be of much benefit to start a high-fiber diet for cancer prevention. Even at that age, it certainly will not hurt, however, to eat high-fiber foods, as regular bowel movements will make the person more comfortable. But it is probably too late for maximum cancer prevention. So eating oats, or any foods high in soluble fiber, may help anyone to avoid constipation, and it may help reduce the risk of cancer and cardiovascular disease by lowering blood lipids. A high-fiber diet will be most effective, however, if maintained for decades or throughout life; the best results occur when the intake of saturated fat and cholesterol is kept low at the same time.

Sugar content is a key component to scrutinize. Nutrient labels list the grams of sugar per one serving size. Therefore, if one serving size is 1 ounce, which is equal to 28 grams, a sweetened breakfast cereal with over 14 grams of sugar in a serving is more than 50% sugar. Some food products with wholesome, healthy image are in fact packed with simple sugars, such as many yogurts and granola bars. For example, one common brand of yogurt I examined consisted of a one-cup serving that contained 42 grams of sugar! That is 1.5 ounces of sugar. In my view, sugar is an underestimated threat to health, and I watch for it very carefully. Sugar often comes as empty calories. That is, an apple has sugar, but it comes with some healthy nutrients and is only 80 calories; although the yogurt above does come with 25% of the daily calcium recommendation, it has 250 calories. Compare that to the mozzarella cheese stick in Figure 17.1, which provides 20% of daily calcium, no sugar, and only 80 calories. Eat two cheese sticks, receive 40% of the recommended calcium intake, and still only consume 160 calories. As we are reminded in the review by Hu and Willett (2002), replacement of saturated fat by carbohydrates increases blood triglycerides and reduces both LDL and HDL cholesterol. So when you read a nutrient label, remember that total carbohydrates include fiber, which is very good—the more the better—and added sugar or high-fructose corn syrup—the less consumed the better.

Daily Reference Values

Daily reference values (DRV) have been established for macronutrients (fat, total carbohydrate, protein), the sources of energy, and for cholesterol, sodium, and potassium, which do not contribute calories (see Figure 17.1). On the label, these values are displayed on the right side under a column labeled %Daily Values (%DV). The value given there represents the percentage of the recommended intake per day for that particular constituent that is provided by one serving of the food. The recommendations are based on an assumed intake of 2000 calories per day and shown in a box at the bottom of the label. That is, if there are 6 grams of fat in one serving and in the lower panel total fat is recommended to be less than 65 grams per day, the serving contains a 9% portion of the recommended daily fat intake.

Labeling and Advertising Claims

We all see the labels that tout "free" this and "low" that. The FDA also stipulates what these words mean by certain standards (FDA 1994). Table 17.2 shows the requirements for describing something as "low" in some compo-

Table 17.1. Calculations for daily reference values (DRV)

Fat based on 30 percent of calories

Saturated fat based on 10 percent of calories

Cholesterol < 300 mg

Sodium < 2,400 mg

Carbohydrate based on 60 percent of calories

Protein based on 10 percent of calories. The DRV for protein applies only to adults and children over 4. "Reference Daily Intake" (RDI) values for protein for special groups have been established.

Fiber based on 11.5 g of fiber per 1,000 calories

Source: FDA (1999).

Table 17.2.   Nutrient content claims

Low	This term can be used for foods that can be eaten frequently without exceeding dietary guidelines for one or more of these components: fat, saturated fat, cholesterol, sodium, and calories. Thus, descriptors are defined as follows:
Low-fat	3 g or less per serving
Low–saturated fat	1 g or less per serving
Low-sodium	140 mg or less per serving
Very low sodium	35 mg or less per serving
Low-cholesterol	20 mg or less and 2 g or less of saturated fat per serving
Low-calorie	40 calories or less per serving

Source: FDA (1999).

nent. If you go to the FDA website as shown, you will find the definitions of the other commonly seen claims.

In summary, food labels are extremely useful for understanding what is in the food you are about to eat, and they can be used to help you strategically include or exclude nutritional components. One key factor is paying attention to serving size and calculating the constituents of interest accordingly. Beware also that low-fat or no-fat often means high-sugar and not necessarily low-calorie.

CHAPTER 18

Alternative Medicine and Fad Diets

Many people are interested in finding alternatives to conventional medicine to cure their health problems. Nowadays there seems to be an endless list of fad diets to choose from, and miracle cures are touted for such serious diseases as diabetes. More and more people are interested in trying out one of those miracle cures that are supposed to be effective and so "natural" or yet another diet that promises "weight loss while eating all you want and not even thinking about exercise." Although there are some documented examples of alternative approaches that work, many, if not most, have dubious or no objective research to assure anyone they are any more effective than placebo and are also safe.

Alternative, Complementary, and Conventional Therapy

For various reasons many people are interested in therapies for a wide range of conditions that do not involve conventional medicine, that is, seeing a physician and using prescription drugs. The reasons for pursuing alternative therapies may include cost, over-the-counter access, or the perception that these compounds are more natural and safer. Somewhat in between alternative therapies and conventional medicine is the complementary approach to medicine. This may take the form, for example, of using dietary supplements in conjunction with more conventional therapies. As an example, Dr. Atkins called part of his practice in New York the Atkins Center for Complementary Medicine because he was using a range of therapies, including dietary supplements. The purpose here is not to describe or debate those issues but rather provide an understanding of some of the important considerations of what so-called natural therapies and cures should include.

Plant-derived medicines, including some forms of modern prescription medicine (digitalis from foxglove plants, tamoxifen from yew tree), have been used effectively for centuries. The use of plant-derived treatments for diabetes goes back as far as 1550 B.C.E. (Gray and Flatt 1997). One example includes the use of cinnamon for improving insulin resistance in diabetes patients. Richard Anderson and colleagues reported results from a small clinical trial involving diabetic patients who consumed 1, 3, or 6 grams of cinnamon per day for 40 days and, for comparison, 3 placebo groups (Khan et al. 2003). Overall, the treated groups had significant decreases in fasting serum glucose (18–29%), triglycerides (23–30%), total cholesterol (12–26%), and LDL cholesterol (7–27%) after 40 days. After 40 days the subjects stopped the cinnamon therapy and by 60 days their values returned to baseline. Throughout the study no changes were found in the placebo groups. This research group also went on to investigate what active compounds in cinnamon seem to provide this action (Anderson et al. 2004). This is an example of at least a limited but objective study of a plant-derived therapy. These types of study are required to develop and pursue validation of any therapy, including a useful plant-derived therapy. These findings also need to be reproduced in larger studies before they can be accepted as a standard of practice. I mentioned the plant-derived stanol-esters (Chapter 15) for reducing cholesterol as another example of a tested therapy, where the active ingredients were known and there had been clinical trials to evaluate safety and effectiveness. It is essential that we evaluate alternative or complementary therapies and learn the active ingredients and if they are they effective and safe.

Some herbal forms of therapy work, but many do not, and some may even cause harm. I recently had a relative contact me for my opinion about a terrific-sounding "cure" for diabetes. A young child in the family has type 1 diabetes mellitus (Chapter 6), and I can fully understand the desire to try anything that sounds this good. This was an herbal combination recently "rediscovered" in Asia. It was now being produced by a little-known company in Canada and being marketed via an 800 telephone number and a website. Since it was herbal, it was being advertised as curative, natural, nontoxic; and for only a few dollars a month, it would cure diabetes.

There are several things I always consider when I hear about new treatments like this. First, the old saying, "if it's too good to be true, it probably is," applies in these cases. There are several inherent problems with these "natural" concoctions. The ingredients, especially the so-called active ingredients, may be highly variable from batch to batch because natural products do not have consistent components. Furthermore, there is often little quality control over production of these concoctions, and inconsistent production results in inconsistent effects and unpredictable toxicities. Since these products are often sold as foods or dietary supplements, the manufacturers are not required by the FDA to prove their effectiveness and nontoxicity. Thus, the natural ingredients may in fact cause some desired action, but this may vary considerably from batch to batch. In many cases no one knows what the active ingredients are, let alone what quantity is present in a given batch.

Another common assumption is that natural ingredients cannot be harmful. This is entirely wrong! There are documented cases of people overdosing on components of "herbal" teas. So these "drugs"—and that is what they are—not only may have no documented benefit, but they could be harmful. Since usually no one has done a careful toxicity study, we may not know of harmful effects until they happen much later. Do not be impressed that a "patent is awarded," as stated on one product I reviewed. Patents provide no credibility to the medical value of a drug or treatment, only that it is a unique combination that cannot legally be made by someone else without the inventor's permission. For the diabetes treatment I was asked about there were published references to studies using it. These publications were in obscure journals that were not credible in my view. The convincing data I would be looking for would include double-blinded studies in dozens to hundreds of diabetic patients who either got the drug or placebo, and neither the patients nor the doctor knew which pill they were getting. After a period of taking the drug, the patients should be evaluated to see who truly improved with a documented rise in insulin level. Was it the drug that provided the therapeutic benefits? A study of that quality would be published in a highly regarded journal, like the *Journal of the American Medical Association*, the *New England Journal of Medicine*, *Journal of Clinical Investigation*, the journal *Diabetes*, or some other major medical journal. Then a major drug company would be buying the rights to this compound in order to market it as a legitimate prescription drug after rigorous safety and efficacy testing. In other words, if this stuff worked as well as was claimed in the magazine advertisement, why is it not sold in the United States? Why has there been no publication of a true clinical trial (double-blinded study) in a major medical journal? How do we know it is harmless, let alone effective? If this is a potentially effective therapy, prove it and prove that it causes no harm.

Recently, a variety of common herbal ingredients, such as St. John's Wort, ginseng, and others, have been shown in controlled studies to have no beneficial effect, as opposed to what was originally claimed. People in clinical trials often got better even when they were given the placebo. These people may have thought they might be getting the new drug, and in their mind it was guaranteed to work, so it must work. That is, they expected to get better, and so they did—the "placebo effect." Diabetes is a terrible disease, and I fully understand wanting to try new treatments that could in fact be a cure. As good as such possibilities sound, a new treatment that has been proven to work will not remain an "alternative" new discovery for long—it will be the welcome new breakthrough being acclaimed by reputable sources.

Diets and the Initial Five-Pound Loss

Diets must also be included in a discussion of alternative therapies. Although what we now call low-carb diets have been known since the nineteenth century—I used the Banting diet as an example in Chapter 13—they have become highly popular over the past 50 years. Unfortunately, it's not commonly recognized that diets have virtually no studies to back up the claims made about them. An overwhelming majority fail over the long term as far as continued practice and maintenance of weight loss that may have occurred. It seems that virtually every diet promises a five-pound weight loss the first week. The initial weight loss is mostly water, not fat, that individuals lose the first week of about any diet regimen. Virtually every diet that reduces calorie intake and stimulates greater use of glycogen, due to a reduction in calories taken in, will result in water loss. Recall that energy is efficiently stored in the body as fat, rather than as glycogen, because glycogen requires storage of a lot of water. Dieting to lose weight as fat is very simple to understand, just hard to do. That is, there must be a reduction in calorie intake, be it fat or carbohydrates, or increased energy expenditure by regular exercise, or some of both for an extended time. A pound of fat has 3,500 calories; a person has to take in 500 fewer calories than usual per day for a week to lose a pound of fat, if activity level remains constant. One approach would be to pass up a piece of chocolate cake and play tennis for 30 minutes. It must be kept in mind, however, that people have different genetic makeups that may drastically affect how easily either side of this energy equation is balanced.

Many alternatives to traditional medical treatments are both available and aggressively advertised. For treatment of diseases of excess fat, these alternatives include "natural" cures and a plethora of diets that promise quick weight loss. Most lack any scientific basis or scrutiny for effectiveness and possible toxicities. They may, however, become popular and make money for entrepreneurs in a society that values initiative, innovation, and success. People want the "next new thing," especially when the peddler of the herb or diet can demonize the men in white coats as the monolithic "medical establishment." At the same time, it is human nature to want to choose the miracle pill over the hard work of making lifelong changes and exercising. It is not surprising that people want to believe they can "melt fat away."

CHAPTER 19

Media Coverage of Health Research

Several times in the last chapter I pointed out that alternative therapies that sound too good to be true should be looked upon with skepticism until supported by solid research. The same is true of conventional therapies. In this chapter I discuss some of the ways biomedical researchers, particularly epidemiologists, try to find cause-and-effect relationships and not just mere "associations" between treatments, like drugs and diets, and human health. If the results of these studies are to do anyone any good, physicians and their patients must learn about them in the professional literature or in the popular media. Occasionally, however, the outcome of a study will be misrepresented in the news, thus causing more confusion among the general public about what is healthy and what is not.

It seems that not a week goes by without some splashy news article reporting that this or that disease is caused by this or that in the diet, and once again mankind is doomed. Despite all the doomsayers, the people of western civilization currently are enjoying the longest lifespan ever. In 1900, the average expected lifespan for white males was only 46.6 years. By 2002, that had increased to 75.1 (National Center for Health Statistics 2005). A major contributor to the lower average lifespan in 1900 was the high rate of infant mortality. Many families would produce four or five children, but only two might survive to adulthood. But middle-aged people are living longer now as well. Today, despite a rapidly increasing rate of obesity and diabetes in children and adults, the average American can look forward to living longer than ever before.

In this chapter, I want to examine several issues about understanding medical research, how researchers try to determine causes and effects in disease processes, and how these cause-and-effect relationships are different from two events simply occurring at the same time. Events that happen to occur at the same time often represent an association, not cause and effect. For example, researchers might collect data on a population of people who have a high rate of fatal heart attacks. They find that a majority of those fatalities had very high blood cholesterol concentrations—also that a majority drove pick-up trucks. The high blood cholesterol concentrations and heart attacks may have a cause-and-effect relationship, whereas driving a pick-up truck is merely an association with fatal heart attacks. Furthermore, I want to explore how clinical trials of human disease processes and treatments are used to determine true causes to the best of our ability. Next, I want to describe how researchers and the news media then report their findings. We the public need to have an eye for results that indicate a meaningless association, even though they make an attention-grabbing headline, rather than a documented cause-and-effect relationship.

Cause and Effect in Disease Processes

One of the biggest challenges in disease research is determining cause and effect, in contrast to observing a whole series of events that simply happen in the process of a disease. What may be even more difficult is to determine whether a new medicine or treatment helps reduce or prevent disease. First of all, it may be unclear as to which event is the cause and which is the effect. Does obesity cause insulin resistance or does insulin resistance cause obesity? First impressions may tell us one thing, but in reality it may be the other way around. The only way to determine which is the cause and which is the effect is to follow prospectively the entire series of events leading up to a disease occurring. Researchers can then witness which came first, "the chicken or the egg." This requires careful experiments that control for each variable that may be involved and that allow researchers to remove or change one variable at a time to test whether it makes a difference in the outcome. A very useful approach many times is the use of animal models of human disease. Eventually, however, after the best estimate has been made in animal models, researchers may use epidemiological studies and clinical trials in human beings to reach the final best conclusion.

Drinking Red Wine and Preventing Heart Attacks

One current item in health news illustrates what I mean by determining true causal relationships. Does wine drinking help prevent cardiovascular disease? There is no doubt that excessive alcohol intake—be it wine, beer, or hard liquor—is not healthy in any way. But how about drinking one or two glasses of wine a day? The idea that wine is good for your heart came to be known as the French paradox because, although the French population, especially in the southern Mediterranean area, does not necessarily eat the low-fat diet often believed to be healthy for hearts, it does have significantly lower rates of cardiovascular disease than other populations. One factor that became evident was that the French on average drank more red wine than the other populations. Is this truly a causal relationship? Does drinking red wine (cause) lead to a healthier heart (effect)?

Several possible mechanisms have been proposed and studies conducted that very well could account for the benefits of drinking red wine. First, folk who drink red wine seem to have increased HDL and lower LDL cholesterol. This may be a direct effect of the alcohol. Second, red wine has a high amount of flavonoids—chemicals that act as anti-oxidants, as vitamin E does—and this could help improve heart health. Flavonoids would give red wine an advantage over white wines or other alcohol-containing drinks. Maybe there really is a cause-and-effect relationship here and we should all pour ourselves a glass of red wine to celebrate. Cheers!

Then other studies were reported. Multiple studies showed that it did not matter what form the alcohol came in—red wine, white wine, beer, or gin—people who had a low to moderate alcohol intake seemed to have this heart health advantage. Then the report came out that, no, there are definite advantages to the anti-oxidant effect, and not only red wine has this advantage, but dark beers have it as well. Then there was the report that simply drinking grape juice had the same advantages. Other reports described positive effects from the alcohol on clotting mechanisms that reduced risk of heart disease. Other reports said that red wine has nothing to do with it; it is simply that people who drink red wine in moderation are the same people who exercise and watch their calorie intake. That is, there is no cause-and-effect relationship at all between drinking red wine and having healthy hearts; it just happened that drinking red wine was more common in people who do a variety of things that turn out to be good for the heart. Some researchers call these type of relationships "epiphenomena." Finally, people who eat the "Mediterranean diet" also tend to consume a lot of olive oil, which is high in monounsaturated fats, which in turn help to increase HDL and lower LDL cholesterol concentrations.

The problem is, there are way too many variables changing at the same time to make clear that one of them is causing the effect of heart disease prevention. So what we end up with are several possible causes (red wine, alcohol alone, olive oil, exercise, etc.) and effects of interest (better blood lipids, decreased heart disease). We look for some answers through epidemiology, the study of disease patterns in populations rather than in individuals. In many studies nothing is actively done to the participants except to collect information from them concerning disease and whatever factor is being investigated. It is very difficult to determine cause and effect in human subjects because not only are so many environmental variables involved—diet, exercise, drinking and smoking habits, drug use, and more—but there is so much genetic diversity in the human population that in many cases the same variable will have different effects even when other factors are held constant. Furthermore, there is often great skepticism about what people say when they are asked what they eat and drink. Let's go back to the example of drinking red wine. What if a study is done in a particular area of France where an allele that helps prevent heart disease is common among the population? No matter how reliable the information obtained on drinking red wine, exercise, and olive oil, will the study be able to determine their influence on cardiovascular disease? The protective effect may come from the genetic characteristics, not the diet, of the participants.

Taking into account the observational studies and proposed mechanisms of action, many researchers involved directly in these studies agree that there may be some direct, positive, long-term benefit of low to moderate alcohol intake, but most are not recommending drinking to raise HDL concentrations and reduce the risk of heart disease. Even Gerald Reaven, who named syndrome X (Chapter 5), has convincing data showing that low to moderate alcohol intake increases insulin sensitivity. He says in his book (Reaven, Strom, and Fox 2000) that although there have been strong indications that drinking some alcohol seems to have heart health benefits, no one has shown that nondrinkers will enjoy significant health benefits if they start drinking. Willett (2001) says the same thing.

Clinical Trials

In order for a drug to be approved by the FDA for the patient market, it must be shown to be effective at a given dose for a given disease or condition, and any side effects must also be determined. Studies must have been done that determine whether the "cause" is the drug and the "effect" is successful treatment of the disease. There are still a large number of variables to contend with, such as age, sex, genetics, and so on, and the only way to assess the true effect of the drug is to test it in very large numbers of people. For example, clinical trials attempting to establish efficacy of a drug on preventing a second heart attack may require the participation of more than 10,000 individuals to find significant results.

In addition to the physical factors being studied is another variable with strong influence, and that one is psychological. Psychological factors may pertain to the patient taking the test drug, as well as to the researcher observing the outcomes of the test drug. The best studies are done when neither the patient nor the researchers know who is getting the real drug and who is getting the placebo. This type of study is called double-blind. Sometimes the placebo is hard to mask, but the best studies are those done where there will be no inherent bias toward either the study group or the control group. Many studies have shown that if people expect a certain result, they can strongly influence the outcome. This can also happen on the side of the observers, who, if they really want the new drug to work, may be more generous in scoring positive outcomes for the patients getting the drug and tend to overlook any side effects. As for the subjects of a study, the "placebo effect" is well known: a patient who thinks he is getting the new drug, but gets a placebo instead, feels much better anyway. Thus, it is better all the way around if neither party knows which treatment the patients are getting and if all patients realize they have an equal chance of getting the real drug or the placebo.

A major way that researchers deal with the problem of differences in results due to sex, age, and genetics is to require that the subjects fit a prescribed set of criteria. For example, if researchers want to test the effectiveness of a new drug that may lower blood cholesterol and heart attack rates in a group of people, do they simply enroll all people who see cardiologists? This is probably not a good idea. A person who has already had a heart attack may be a very different "experimental subject" than a person who is being followed for possible heart disease (because his lipids are high and he has a strong family history of heart disease) but has not had a heart attack. By enrolling only people who fit a prescribed set of criteria, researchers hope that the conclusions drawn will apply to all people with those specific characteristics (although they may also apply to others). Furthermore, the people enrolled should be randomly assigned to treatment and control groups. For many years, most studies included only adult men, often only white men. The results of such studies, however, may or may not apply to other groups in the population, especially children. Now the National Institutes of Health insist that all groups be represented in studies; any exclusion of groups must be justified in detail. For some studies, however, there may be a limited number of patients from particular racial groups who have certain diseases. For example, sickle-cell disease is found predominantly in blacks, and cystic fibrosis predominantly in whites.

Studies May Be Stopped Early

Sometimes a study will be stopped before the planned end date. If the treatment group is clearly benefiting from the treatment, the results may not be held back for even more proof. If either the treatment or the control group is being harmed, the study is stopped for their safety. Before a study begins, the philosophy is "the researchers really do not know if this drug will improve things or not," so ethically the researchers are not depriving the control group of possible benefits by giving out placebos. There is an oversight committee, also known as the Data Safety and Monitoring Board, for each study that is independent of the researchers. The committee members know who is getting the drug and who is getting the placebo and reviews the data periodically throughout the study. If, halfway through the planned study, the oversight committee is persuaded either that the drug is clearly working better than the placebo or that an undesirable outcome is associated with the drug, it will stop the study so that the control group can be given the drug or so that both groups are protected from harm. Many studies, however, need literally years of following thousands of patients to get clear results.

Public Effects of Clinical Trials

If the results of a study, good or bad, are reported in the news, the drug company's stock price gains or loses accordingly. Drug companies invest around $500 million and decades of development time to bring a new drug to market. As you can imagine, good or bad news has a tremendous impact on the company. Drug development is a very risky business. What is most important in my mind is that we know for certain that a drug will be safe and effective against disease. Regulatory oversight is supposed to ensure that this is so. Nevertheless, things can get out of hand when public perception and stock prices are added to the mix. At this point careful oversight of conflicts of interest is crucial. Review boards at research institutions, like universities, where studies are done provide oversight to protect human subjects and assure they give informed consent to participate in the study. Studies must be done under full disclosure: it must be clear who is paying whom to carry out the research. It is also important that researchers not hold press conferences to announce premature results, which can affect stock prices no matter how carefully phrased the "tentative" results are explained.

Intentionally or not, the news media sometimes misrepresents results of clinical trials, adding to the public's confusion over the risks and benefits of foods, medicines, and other things. A recent example occurred when in a single issue of the *New England Journal of Medicine* two studies reported that high-fiber diets did not prevent recurrence of colorectal adenomas, a precancerous lesion of the colon (Alberts et al. 2000; Schatzkin et al. 2000). What the research articles said was that switching to a high-fiber, low-fat diet did not help prevent recurrence of colorectal adenomas in people who had already had a diagnosis of polyps or precancerous (colorectal adenomas) lesions. In response, the news media reported that high-fiber, low-fat diets are of no help in preventing colon cancer in *anyone*. Note the titles of the original research articles:

- Alberts, D.S., et al. 2000. "Lack of effect of a high-fiber cereal supplement on the *recurrence* of colorectal adenomas." *New England Journal of Medicine* 342: 1156–1162.
- Schatzkin, A., et al. 2000. "Lack of effect of a low-fat, high-fiber diet on the *recurrence* of colorectal adenomas." *New England Journal of Medicine* 342: 1149–1155. [Emphasis is mine.]

Both titles clearly say *recurrence*, meaning that the subjects of the study already had tumors in their colons at the beginning of the study. The point of these studies was to ask whether a dietary change would prevent *return* of the tumors. The headlines in newspapers failed to make this distinction:

- Beil, L. 2000. "Study fails to find evidence that high-fiber, low-fat diet prevents colon cancer." *Dallas Morning News*, April 19 (cover story).
- Vergano, D. 2000. "Diet's role in colon cancer in doubt. Two studies suggest high fiber fails to prevent polyps." *USA Today*, April 20 (cover story).
- Kolata, G. 2000. "Two fiber studies find no benefit for the colon. Surprised

teams detect no cancer protection." *New York Times,* April 20 (cover story).

These headlines strongly imply that high-fiber diets have no beneficial effects in preventing colon cancer at all.

The published reports may sound similar (medical papers versus the newspaper reports), but they are really very different. First, if someone already has precancerous lesions or even malignant transformation of cells ongoing in their colon, it is highly unlikely that switching to a high-fiber diet (or anything else) will prevent the eventual development of colon cancer. The way in which a high-fiber diet might *possibly* help prevent colon cancer is this: eating a high-fiber diet keeps the digested food, which presumably contains the toxic compounds that induce development of cancer, moving rapidly through the intestinal tract. This decreases the time the toxins are present in the body to incite cancer, which may help prevent colon cancer. It takes many years for colon cancer to develop, and a high-fiber diet can be of benefit only if it is followed over the years—not after precancerous changes have already begun to occur. The protective effect was first noticed, by Denis P. Burkitt (of Burkitt's lymphoma fame), in a population in Africa whose diet included a lot of high-fiber vegetables and who had virtually no colon cancer (Burkitt 1971). So it is not surprising that at the late stages of already-developing colon cancer the addition of fiber to the diet did not produce a benefit. This does not mean that a high-fiber diet throughout life will not be beneficial for preventing colon cancer. Researchers are not yet certain that it will, but my point is that there is a big difference between stating that four years of a high-fiber, low-fat diet did not prevent *recurrence* of colorectal adenomas (scientists) and stating that high-fiber, low-fat diets *do not* prevent colon cancer (newspaper headlines). The authors of the *New England Journal of Medicine* articles actually stated in their conclusions that their studies were an attempt to prevent recurrence. Some clarifying details that I have mentioned here are discussed in some of the newspaper articles, but the three headlines present the reader with a foregone conclusion: high fiber is of no benefit in preventing colon cancer. No wonder people are confused about what to eat.

An understanding of cause and effect in disease development and in ways of treating disease is sometimes very difficult to come by. Epidemiological studies and clinical trials of drugs or treatments require large numbers of people who must be unbiased in both their participation and their evaluation. The next time you come across a major claim in the news, make sure that the headline really matches the results. Also consider whether the conclusion is being presented in a professional journal as part of a completed study and is not just a premature release of tentative findings to the popular press.

Glossary

References

Index

Glossary

ACC   Acetyl-CoA carboxylase, the enzyme that produces malonyl-CoA from acetyl-CoA for the synthesis of fatty acids and inhibition of fatty acid oxidation at CPT-1.

acetyl-CoA   A 2-carbon acetyl-residue attached to a coenzyme A; also known as active acetate. Synthesized from glucose if insulin is present, this molecule is used in the production of malonyl-CoA, which is required for fatty acid synthesis. Acetyl-CoA is also the substrate for energy production in the TCA cycle, ketogenesis, and cholesterol synthesis.

acyl-CoA   A fatty acid substrate (having 4 or more carbons) with a coenzyme A attached. Produced from free fatty acids inside cells, acyl-CoA is the form of fatty acid that is ready to be oxidized for production of energy or for storage in triglycerides.

adipocytes   Cells in the adipose tissue that store fats inside a vacuole and secrete essential hormones that affect regulation of feeding behavior, activity level, and metabolic rate.

adipose tissue   Tissue that stores triglycerides and produces hormones such as leptin; also known as body fat. *See* adipocytes.

allele   A sequence variant of a gene at a given location (locus). Each individual has two alleles for each gene, one inherited from the mother and one from the father. A wild-type (normal) allele has the sequence found in the majority of the population. Variant alleles are found in much smaller proportions of the population and may be passed to offspring, just as normal alleles are.

apolipoproteins   Large proteins composing the exterior of lipoproteins that serve as targets for receptor molecules in cell membranes and provide for transport of water-insoluble lipids in the bloodstream.

ATP   Adenosine triphosphate stores the chemical energy that living organisms require for biological functions. Energy is stored in the chemical bonds of the ATP molecule and is released when these bonds are broken during chemical reactions.

β-oxidation   Another term for fatty acid oxidation. Through a series of chemical steps, long-chain fatty acids are broken down into smaller and smaller acyl–Coenzyme A molecules two carbon units at a time, producing acetyl-CoA. Acetyl-CoA is used for further energy production.

BMI   Body mass index is a simple estimate of body "fatness," calculated as a person's weight in kilograms divided by height in meters squared.

carbohydrates   Molecules with the general form $(CH_2O)_x$ with $x \geq 3$ that make up the substances known as sugars and starches.

CCK   Cholecystokinin, a peptide produced in the small intestine that influences satiety and suppresses appetite.

cholesterol   A sterol compound used by the body for cell membrane structure, as well as a precursor for steroid hormones. When in excess, cholesterol is associated with cardiovascular disease.

chylomicron   A large, triglyceride-rich lipoprotein that carries the dietary-derived lipids, including cholesterol, in the bloodstream.

CPT-1   Carnitine palmitoyltransferase-1, an enzyme that regulates the influx of fatty acids into mitochondria for fatty acid oxidation. It is therefore known as the "gatekeeper" of β-oxidation.

CPT-2   Carnitine palmitoyltransferase-2, an enzyme inside the mitochondrion that converts acylcarnitines back to acyl-CoA.

diabetes mellitus, type 1   Previously known as insulin-dependent diabetes mellitus.

diabetes mellitus, type 2   Previously known as noninsulin-dependent diabetes mellitus.

enzyme   A protein that serves as a catalyst for biochemical reactions in the body.

ester   Compound molecule formed by attachment of an acid and an alcohol. The cholesterol that is carried in blood by lipoproteins is predominantly esterified cholesterol (i.e., a cholesterol molecule with a fatty acid attached).

ETF   Electron transport flavoprotein, a co-factor needed in acyl-CoA dehydrogenase reactions of fatty acid oxidation.

expressivity   The strength or weakness with which a particular genotype affects individuals carrying the same alleles. The effect may vary depending on which alleles of other genes a person has inherited or on environmental influences.

FADH₂   Flavin dinucleotide-reduced, derived from the B-vitamin riboflavin.

FAO   Fatty acid oxidation. *See* β-oxidation.

fatty acid   An acid (i.e., a molecule with the capacity to release a hydrogen ion, or H^+) made up of a hydrocarbon chain with a carboxyl group (—COOH) on one end. Fatty acids are broken down in the body's cells for energy production. *See* β-oxidation.

FFA/NEFA   Free fatty acid, or its synonym nonesterified fatty acid. In this form, fatty acids are insoluble in water and must be associated with the protein albumin for transport in the bloodstream.

FH Familial hypercholesterolemia, an inherited disease caused by a genetic deficiency of LDL receptors and characterized by extremely high concentrations of LDL cholesterol in the blood.

fiber A form of carbohydrate that cannot be digested and absorbed into the body for use as fuel or fat storage.

fibrates A class of drugs used to lower blood triglycerides by activating PPAR-α, thus increasing fatty acid oxidation and reducing VLDL triglyceride.

fructose A sugar with the same chemical formula as glucose, $C_6H_{12}O_6$, but with a different configuration.

gene A segment of DNA in the genome that contains a molecular sequence ultimately encoding for a protein or RNA and the requisite regulatory elements.

gene product The protein or RNA produced when a gene is activated.

genotype The alleles of genes for a particular trait inherited by an individual.

ghrelin A peptide produced in the stomach that stimulates appetite.

GLP-1 Glucagon-like peptide-1, which is produced in the small intestine and suppresses appetite.

glucagon Hormone secreted by the pancreas that stimulates the breakdown of glycogen into glucose and triglycerides into fatty acids and glycerol. It also stimulates gluconeogenesis and ketogenesis.

gluconeogenesis The process of synthesizing glucose from noncarbohydrate sources, such as amino acids, glycerol, or propionate.

glucose A sugar, $C_6H_{12}O_6$, that is a major energy source for the body and is transported by blood to cells for energy or for storage as fat.

glycemic index Index relating on average a person's blood glucose response to eating a certain food, where 50 grams of glucose or white bread equals 1.

glycerol A product of glucose metabolism, glycerol is used to connect 3 fatty acids in a triglyceride molecule.

glycogen The storage form of glucose in the body. In the liver, it is broken down into glucose and released into the bloodstream, but inside cells it is both broken down into and put back together from glucose-6-phosphate.

glycogenolysis The breakdown of glycogen into glucose, a process that is initiated by an increase in epinephrine or glucagon.

glycolipids Lipids with both fatty acid moieties (functioning parts) and carbohydrate moieties.

glycolysis The breakdown of glucose to form pyruvate.

HbA$_{1c}$ Normal hemoglobin A found in red blood cells with a glucose attached. The fraction of hemoglobin-A$_{1c}$ increases in diabetic patients.

HDL High-density lipoprotein, called the "good cholesterol" because it carries cholesterol to the liver for disposal from the body.

HELLP   A syndrome characterized by hypertension, elevated liver enzymes, and low platelets. It is found in mothers with fetuses affected by LCHAD deficiency.

hepatocyte   Cells in the liver that are specialized for various metabolic functions.

HLA   Human leukocyte antigen.

HMG-CoA   3-Hydroxy-3-methyl-glutaryl-CoA is derived from acetoacetyl-CoA with acetyl-CoA and converted into mevalonate, the rate-limiting step of cholesterol synthesis (cytosolic) or acetoacetate in ketogenesis (mitochondrial).

hormone   Substance produced by cells in the body and secreted into the bloodstream for the regulation of metabolic processes.

hydrogenated fat   Usually polyunsaturated or monounsaturated vegetable fat that has been treated with hydrogen gas in order to form *trans* fatty acids and make the fat hard.

hyperglycemia   Elevated blood glucose concentrations.

hyperinsulinemia   Elevated blood insulin concentrations.

hypertension   High blood pressure.

hypertriglyceridemia   Elevated blood triglyceride concentrations.

inborn errors of metabolism   Inherited diseases of metabolism usually due to enzyme deficiency.

insulin   Hormone that stimulates glucose uptake by tissues and synthesis of glycerol and acetyl-CoA from glucose, promotes for the synthesis of fatty acids, and inhibits fatty acid oxidation.

insulin receptor   The receptor on cellular membranes that interacts with insulin and mediates the downstream effects of insulin action, such as glucose uptake.

insulin resistance   A condition in which increased amounts of insulin are needed to act on a cell to get the "normal" response, such as glucose uptake.

ketoacidosis   A dangerous condition of excessive ketone bodies in the blood.

ketone body   A by-product of fat metabolism in the liver that is used as an energy source in other body tissues.

ketosis   Elevation of ketone bodies in the blood (and urine) that occurs when blood glucose levels are low (and therefore unavailable for use as energy).

LCAD   Long-chain acyl-CoA dehydrogenase, an enzyme of the fatty acid β-oxidation pathway.

LCHAD   Long-chain hydroxyacyl-CoA dehydrogenase, an enzyme of the fatty acid β-oxidation pathway.

LDL   Low-density lipoprotein derived from VLDL and containing a high proportion of cholesterol ester. Also known as the "bad cholesterol" because this cholesterol is being delivered to cells.

leptin   Hormone involved in feeding behavior by either inhibiting chemical signals that stimulate food intake or activating signals that suppress food intake.

lipases   Enzymes that break down lipids.

lipids Natural substances that include fatty acids, or their derivates, and cholesterol. All of these compounds are insoluble in water.

lipodystrophy A pathologic condition of abnormal distribution of body fat, which may include loss of fat and excess deposition fat at the same time.

lipolysis The process of breaking down triglycerides into constituent parts, such as fatty acids and glycerol; the term usually refers to the breakdown of triglycerides stored in the adipose tissue.

lipoproteins Protein-lipid complexes that form particles that transport lipids in the blood.

locus (*pl.,* loci) A particular location in the genome where a gene or a specific DNA segment resides.

malonyl-CoA A product of glucose metabolism, consisting of a 3-carbon fatty acid precursor attached to a coenzyme A. Malonyl-CoA provides the 2-carbon units needed to synthesize fatty acids with the loss of a CO_2.

MCAD Medium-chain acyl-CoA dehydrogenase, an enzyme of the fatty acid β-oxidation pathway.

metabolic syndrome A complex syndrome characterized by some or all of the following: insulin resistance, hypertension, hyperinsulinemia, hypertriglyceridemia, low HDL, obesity, and abnormal clotting of blood.

mitochondrion A structure in the cellular cytoplasm where oxidation and energy production take place.

NADH Nicotinamide adenine dinucleotide-reduced, which is derived from the B-vitamin niacin.

NAFLD Nonalcoholic fatty liver disease, often considered a predecessor condition to NASH.

NASH Nonalcoholic steatohepatitis, a severe fatty change and inflammation of the liver.

necrosis Cell death.

oxidation In general, a chemical reaction with a transfer of electrons to an acceptor protein (e.g., ETF) or oxygen. Both fatty acids and glucose are oxidized for energy production.

penetrance The proportion of individuals in a population with a genotype known to cause a trait. If all individuals show the trait associated with that genotype, this is known as complete penetrance. If some individuals have the genotype but do not show the trait, penetrance is said to be incomplete. The severity of the trait is not considered; *see* expressivity.

phenotype The physical characteristics of an individual (such as eye color or high or low concentration of lipids in the blood) that depend entirely or only in part on the individual's genotype.

phospholipids Lipids that have a structure like triglycerides (3 fatty acids held together by a glycerol) but on one of the three positions a phosphate with a variable moiety is attached that gives the lipid a charge and specific properties.

placebo   A fake medicine given in clinical trials so that the participants, both those receiving and those not receiving the actual medicine, do not know whether they are being treated.

polymorphism   Literally means "many forms," here referring to various DNA sequences at a given locus.

POMC   Pro-opiomelanocortin is the precursor to several peptide hormones made in the brain, including α-melanocyte-stimulating hormone, which functions to suppress food intake when activated by leptin.

PPAR   Peroxisomal proliferator activated receptor, a transcription factor that mediates the effects of fatty acids, fibrates, and glitazone-type drugs.

protein   A large molecular compound consisting of a sequence of amino acids.

receptor   A molecule in the membrane of a cell that interacts with molecules on other cells or with portions of molecules carried by the blood. This interaction will stimulate or inhibit a reaction between the cells or between the cell and the outside molecule.

SCAD   Short-chain acyl-CoA dehydrogenase, an enzyme of the fatty acid β-oxidation pathway.

SIDS   Sudden Infant Death Syndrome.

SNP   Single nucleotide polymorphism.

SREBP   Sterol-response element binding protein, a transcription factor that regulates cholesterol and fatty acid synthesis.

statins   A group of drugs that function as inhibitors of HMG-CoA reductase, a rate-limiting step of cholesterol synthesis.

sterol   An alcohol (i.e., a compound molecule with an —OH group) with a characteristic 4-ring steroid nucleus. Cholesterol is one of many types of sterols.

syndrome X   An early name for metabolic syndrome or insulin resistance syndrome.

TCA cycle   Tricarboxylic acid cycle, also known as the Krebs cycle, the metabolic pathway in mitochondria that releases energy stored in chemical bonds for use by the body.

triacylglycerol   A synonym for triglyceride.

triglyceride   A common storage form of lipid, composed of three fatty acids attached to a glycerol backbone.

TZD   A drug group used to treat insulin resistance; also known as the thiazolidinediones or the glitazones.

VLCAD   Very long-chain acyl-CoA dehydrogenase, an enzyme of the fatty acid β-oxidation pathway.

VLDL   Very low-density lipoprotein, which is produced predominantly by the liver and contains a high proportion of triglycerides.

References

Introduction: Lessons from a Mouse

Coleman, D. L. 1978. "*Obese* and *Diabetes:* Two Mutant Genes Causing Diabetes-Obesity Syndromes in Mice." *Diabetologia* 14: 141–148.

Schuler, A. M., and P. A. Wood. 2002. "Mouse Models for Disorders of Mitochondrial Fatty Acid β-Oxidation." *Institute for Laboratory Animal Research Journal, National Academy of Sciences* 43: 57–65.

Wood, P. A. 2004. "Genetically Modified Mouse Models for Disorders of Fatty Acid Metabolism: Pursuing the Nutrigenomics of Insulin Resistance and Type 2 Diabetes." *Nutrition* 20: 121–126.

Zhang, Y., R. Proenca, M. Maffei, M. Barone, L. Leopold, and J. M. Friedman. 1994. "Positional Cloning of the Mouse *Obese* Gene and Its Human Homologue." *Nature* 372: 425–432.

1. The Burden of Obesity

Barsh, G. S., I. S. Farooqi, and S. O'Rahilly. 2000. "Genetics of Body-Weight Regulation." *Nature* 404: 644–651.

Campfield, L. A., F. J. Smith, and P. Burn. 1998. "Strategies and Potential Molecular Targets for Obesity Treatment." *Science* 280: 1383–1387.

Comuzzie, A. G., and D. B. Allison. 1998. "The Search for Human Obesity Genes." *Science* 280: 1374–1377.

Flier, J. F. 2004. "Obesity Wars: Molecular Progress Confronts an Expanding Epidemic." *Cell* 116: 337–350.

Lara-Castro, C., R. L. Weinsier, G. R. Hunter, and R. Desmond. 2002. "Visceral Adipose Tissue in Women: Longitudinal Study of the Effects of Fat Gain, Time, and Race." *Obesity Research* 10: 868–874.

National Diabetes Education Program (NDEP). 2004. "An Update on Type 2 Diabetes in Youth from the National Diabetes Education Program, 2004." *Pediatrics* 114: 259–263.

Pi-Sunyer, F. X. 2003. "A Clinical View of the Obesity Problem." *Science* 299: 859–860.

Rocchini, A. P. 2002. "Childhood Obesity and a Diabetes Epidemic." *New England Journal of Medicine* 346: 854–855.

Rosenbloom, A. L., R. S. Young, J. R. Joe, and W. E. Winter. 1999. "Emerging Epidemic of Type 2 Diabetes in Youth." *Diabetes Care* 22: 345–354.

Strauss, R. S., and H. A. Pollack. 2001. "Epidemic Increase in Childhood Overweight, 1986–1998." *Journal of the American Medical Association* 286: 2845–2848.

Sturm, R. 2002. "The Effects of Obesity, Smoking and Drinking on Medical Problems and Costs." *Health Affairs* 21: 245–253.

Wickelgren, I. 1998. "Obesity: How Big a Problem?" *Science* 280: 1364–1367.

Woods, S. C., R. J. Seeley, D. Porte, and M. W. Schwartz. 1998. "Signals That Regulate Food Intake and Energy Homeostasis." *Science* 280: 1378–1383.

Zhang, Y., R. Proenca, M. Maffei, M. Barone, L. Leopold, and J. M. Friedman. 1994. "Positional Cloning of the Mouse *Obese* Gene and Its Human Homologue." *Nature* 372: 425–432.

2. Testing for Silent Diseases

Matsuzawa, Y. 1997. "Pathophysiology and Molecular Mechanisms of Visceral Fat Syndrome: The Japanese Experience." *Diabetes/Metabolism Reviews* 13: 3–13.

Reaven, G., T. K. Strom, and B. Fox. 2000. *Syndrome X: The Silent Killer, the New Heart Disease Risk.* New York: Simon and Schuster.

4. Disorders of Excess Cholesterol and Triglycerides

Bloch, K. 1965. "The Biological Synthesis of Cholesterol." *Science* 15: 19–28.

Brown, M. S., and J. L. Goldstein. 1997. "The SREBP Pathway: Regulation of Cholesterol Metabolism by Proteolysis of a Membrane Bound Transcription Factor." *Cell* 89: 331–340.

Dietschy, J. M. 1997. "Theoretical Considerations of What Regulates Low-Density-Lipoprotein and High-Density-Lipoprotein Cholesterol." *American Journal of Clinical Nutrition* 65 (suppl): 1581S–1589S.

Durrington, P. 2003. "Dyslipidaemia." *Lancet* 362: 717–731.

Goldstein, J. L., H. H. Hobbs, and M. S. Brown. 2001. "Familial Hypercholesterolemia." In C. R. Scriver, A. L. Beaudet, W. S. Sly, D. Valle, B. Childs, K. W. Kinzler, and B. Vogelstein, eds., *The Metabolic and Molecular Bases of Inherited Disease*, 2863–2913. New York: McGraw-Hill.

Gotto, A. M. 1999. *Contemporary Diagnosis and Management of Lipid Disorders.* Newtown, PA: Handbooks in Healthcare.

Grundy, S. M., E. H. Ahrens, and J. Davignon. 1969. "The Interaction of Cholesterol

Absorption and Cholesterol Synthesis in Man." *Journal of Lipid Research* 10: 304–315.

Kane, J. P., and R. J. Havel. 2001. "Disorders of Biogenesis and Secretion of Lipoproteins Containing the B Lipoproteins." In C. R. Scriver, A. L. Beaudet, W. S. Sly, D. Valle, B. Childs, K. W. Kinzler, and B. Vogelstein, eds., *The Metabolic and Molecular Bases of Inherited Disease,* 2717–2752. New York: McGraw-Hill.

Mayes, P. A. 2000. "Lipid Transport and Storage." In R. K. Murray, D. K. Granner, P. A. Mayes, V. W. Rodwell, eds., *Harper's Biochemistry,* 268–284. New York: McGraw-Hill.

National Cholesterol Education Program (NCEP). 2004. "Implications of Recent Clinical Trials for the National Cholesterol Education Program Adult Treatment Panel III Guidelines." Accessed on Nov. 11, 2004, at www.nhlbi.nih.gov/guidelines/cholesterol/atp3upd04.htm.

5. Insulin Resistance and Metabolic Syndrome

Browning, J. D., and J. D. Horton. 2004. "Molecular Mediators of Hepatic Steatosis and Liver Injury." *Journal of Clinical Investigation* 114: 147–152.

Expert Committee on the Diagnosis and Classification of Diabetes Mellitus. 2003. "Follow-Up Report on the Diagnosis of Diabetes Mellitus." *Diabetes Care* 26: 3160–3167.

Ford, E. S., W. H. Giles, and W. H. Dietz. 2002. "Prevalence of the Metabolic Syndrome among US Adults." *Journal of the American Medical Association* 287: 356–359.

Matsuzawa, Y. 1997. "Pathophysiology and Molecular Mechanisms of Visceral Fat Syndrome: The Japanese Experience." *Diabetes/Metabolism Reviews* 13: 3–13.

Petersen, K. F., D. Befroy, S. Dufour, J. Dziura, C. Ariyan, D. L. Rothman, L. DiPietro, G. W. Cline, and G. I. Shulman. 2003. "Mitochondrial Dysfunction in the Elderly: Possible Role in Insulin Resistance." *Science* 300: 1140–1142.

Petersen, K. F., S. Dufour, D. Befroy, R. Garcia, and G. I. Shulman. 2004. "Impaired Mitochondrial Activity in the Insulin-Resistant Offspring of Patients with Type 2 Diabetes." *New England Journal of Medicine* 350: 664–671.

Reaven, G. M. 1988. "Role of Insulin Resistance in Human Disease." *Diabetes* 37: 1595–1607.

Reaven, G. M., T. K. Strom, and B. Fox. 2000. *Syndrome X: The Silent Killer, the New Heart Disease Risk.* New York: Simon and Schuster.

Shulman, G. I. 2000. "Insulin Resistance. Cellular Mechanisms of Insulin Resistance." *Journal of Clinical Investigation* 106: 171–176.

6. Type 1 and Type 2 Diabetes

Brix, A. E., A. Elgavish, T. R. Nagy, B. A. Gower, W. J. Rhead, and P. A. Wood. 2002. "Evaluation of Liver Fatty Acid Oxidation in the Leptin Deficient *Obese* Mouse." *Molecular Genetics and Metabolism* 75: 219–226.

Eisenbarth, G. S., A. G. Ziegler, and P. A. Colman. 1994. "Pathogenesis of Insulin-Dependent (Type 1) Diabetes Mellitus." In C. R. Kahn and G. C. Weir, eds., *Joslin's Diabetes Mellitus*, 216–239. Philadelphia: Lea and Febiger.

Kurtz, D. M., L. Tian, B. A. Gower, T. R. Nagy, C. A. Pinkert, and P. A. Wood. 2000. "Transgenic Studies of Fatty Acid Oxidation Gene Expression in Nonobese Diabetic Mice." *Journal of Lipid Research* 41: 2063–2070.

McGarry, J. D. 1992. "What If Minkowski Had Been Ageusic? An Alternative Angle on Diabetes." *Science* 258: 766–770.

Taylor, S. I. 1995. "Diabetes mellitus." In C. R. Scriver, A. L. Beaudet, W. S. Sly, and D. Valle, eds., *The Metabolic and Molecular Bases of Inherited Disease*, 843–896. New York: McGraw-Hill.

7. The Energy Equation

Rosenbaum, M., R. Leibel, and J. Hirsch. 1997. "Obesity." *New England Journal of Medicine* 337: 396–407.

8. Making and Storing Fat

Wakil, S. J. 1989. "Fatty Acid Synthase, a Proficient Multifunctional Enzyme." *Biochemistry* 28: 4523–4530.

9. Burning Fat in the Cell

Greville, G. D., and P. K. Tubbs. 1968. "The Catabolism of Long-Chain Fatty Acids in Mammalian Tissues." *Essays in Biochemistry* 4: 155–212.

10. Single-Gene Disorders of Lipid Metabolism

Brown, M. S., and J. L. Goldstein. 1997. "The SREBP Pathway: Regulation of Cholesterol Metabolism by Proteolysis of a Membrane Bound Transcription Factor." *Cell* 89: 331–340.

Brunzell, J. D., and S. S. Deeb. 2001. "Familial Lipoprotein Lipase Deficiency, Apo C-II Deficiency, and Hepatic Lipase Deficiency." In C. R. Scriver, A. L. Beaudet, W. S. Sly, D. Valle, B. Childs, K. W. Kinzler, and B. Vogelstein, eds., *The Metabolic and Molecular Bases of Inherited Disease*, 2789–2816. New York: McGraw-Hill.

Butgereit, B. "Fatal Illness Fears." *Birmingham News*, January 18, 1992, A1.

Cox, K. B., D. A. Hamm, D. S. Millington, D. Matern, J. Vockley, P. Rinaldo, C. A. Pinkert, W. J. Rhead, J. R. Lindsey, and P. A. Wood. 2001. "Gestational, Pathologic, and Biochemical Differences between Very Long Chain Acyl-CoA Dehydrogenase Deficiency and Long-Chain Acyl-CoA Dehydrogenase Deficiency in the Mouse." *Human Molecular Genetics* 10: 2069–2077.

Goldstein, J. L., H. H. Hobbs, and M. S. Brown. 2001. "Familial Hypercholesterolemia." In C. R. Scriver, A. L. Beaudet, W. S. Sly, D. Valle, B. Childs, K. W. Kinzler, and B.

Vogelstein, eds., *The Metabolic and Molecular Bases of Inherited Disease*, 2863–2913. New York: McGraw-Hill.

Gotto, A. M. 1999. *Contemporary Diagnosis and Management of Lipid Disorders.* Newtown, PA: Handbooks in Healthcare.

Guerra, C., R. A. Koza, K. Walsh, D. M. Kurtz, P. A. Wood, and L. P. Kozak. 1998. "Abnormal Nonshivering Thermogenesis in Mice with Inherited Defects of Fatty Acid Oxidation." *Journal of Clinical Investigation* 102: 1724–1731.

Ibdah, J. A., M. J. Bennett, P. Rinaldo, Y. Zhao, B. Gibson, H. F. Sims, and A. W. Strauss. 1999. "A Fetal Fatty Acid Oxidation Disorder as a Cause of Liver Disease in Pregnant Women." *New England Journal of Medicine* 340: 1723–1731.

Kane, J. P., and R. J. Havel. 2001. "Disorders of Biogenesis and Secretion of Lipoproteins Containing B Apolipoproteins." In C. R. Scriver, A. L. Beaudet, W. S. Sly, D. Valle, B. Childs, K. W. Kinzler, B. Vogelstein, eds., *The Metabolic and Molecular Bases of Inherited Disease*, 2717–2752. New York: McGraw-Hill.

Kurtz, D. M., P. Rinaldo, W. J. Rhead, L. Tian, D. S. Millington, J. Vockley, D. A. Hamm, A. E. Brix, J. R. Lindsey, C. A. Pinkert, W. E. O'Brien, and P. A. Wood. 1998. "Targeted Disruption of Mouse Long-Chain Acyl-CoA Dehydrogenase Reveals Crucial Roles for Fatty Acid Oxidation." *Proceedings of National Academy Sciences (USA)* 95: 15592–15597.

Mahley, R. W., and S. C. Rall, Jr. 2001. "Type III Hyperlipoproteinemia (Dysbetalipoproteinemia): The Role of Apolipoprotein E in Normal and Abnormal Lipoprotein Metabolism." In C. R. Scriver, A. L. Beaudet, W. S. Sly, D. Valle, B. Childs, K. W. Kinzler, and B. Vogelstein, eds., *The Metabolic and Molecular Bases of Inherited Disease*, 2835–2862. New York: McGraw-Hill.

Mayes, P. A. 2000. "Cholesterol Synthesis, Transport and Excretion." In R. K. Murray, D. K. Granner, P. A. Mayes, and V. W. Rodwell, eds., *Harper's Biochemistry*, 285–297. New York: McGraw-Hill.

Rader, D. J. 1996. "Genetic Dyslipoproteinemias." In N. Blau, M. Duran, M. E. Blaskovics, eds. *Physician's Guide to the Laboratory Diagnosis of Metabolic Diseases.* 407–418. London: Chapman and Hall.

Roe, C. R., and J. Ding. 2001. "Mitochondrial Fatty Acid Oxidation Disorders." In C. R. Scriver, A. L. Beaudet, W. S. Sly, D. Valle, B. Childs, K. W. Kinzler, and B. Vogelstein, eds., *The Metabolic and Molecular Bases of Inherited Disease*, 2297–2326. New York: McGraw-Hill.

Wood, P. A. 1999. "Defects in Mitochondrial β-Oxidation of Fatty Acids." *Current Opinion in Lipidology*, 10: 107–112.

11. Multifactorial Genetic Diseases of Lipid Metabolism

Kahn, S. E., and D. Porte. 2001. "β-Cell Dysfunction in Type 2 Diabetes: Pathophysiological and Genetic Bases." In C. R. Scriver, A. L. Beaudet, W. S. Sly, D. Valle, B.

Childs, K. W. Kinzler, and B. Vogelstein, eds., *The Metabolic and Molecular Bases of Inherited Disease*, 1407–1431. New York: McGraw-Hill.

Nussbaum, R. L., R. R. McInnes, and H. F. Williard. 2001. *Genetics in Medicine*, 79–109 and 289–310. Philadelphia: W. B. Saunders.

Roses, A. D. 2000. "Pharmacogenetics and the Practice of Medicine." *Nature* 405: 857–865.

12. Overcoming Genetics and Aging

Baier, L. J., and R. L. Hanson. 2004. "Genetic Studies of the Etiology of Type 2 Diabetes in Pima Indians: Hunting for Pieces of a Complicated Puzzle." *Diabetes* 53: 1181–1186.

Hagan, M. M., P. K. Wauford, P. C. Chandler, L. A. Jarrett, R. J. Rybak, and K. Blackburn. 2002. "A New Animal Model of Binge Eating: Key Synergistic Role of Past Caloric Restriction and Stress." *Physiology and Behavior* 77: 45–54.

Knowler, W. C., D. J. Pettitt, M. F. Saad, and P. H. Bennett. 1990. "Diabetes Mellitus in the Pima Indians: Incidence, Risk Factors and Pathogenesis." *Diabetes/Metabolism Reviews* 6:1–27.

Lee, C. C., J. Z. Kasa-Vuba, and M. A. Supiano. 2004. "Androgenicity and Obesity Are Independently Associated with Insulin Sensitivity in Postmenopausal Women." *Metabolism* 53: 507–512.

Nerbrand, C., J. Lidfeldt, P. Nyberg, B. Schersten, and G. Samsioe. 2004. "Serum Lipids and Lipoproteins in Relation to Endogenous and Exogenous Female Sex Steroids and Age: The Women's Health in the Lund Area (WHILA) Study." *Maturitas* 48: 161–169.

Petersen, K. F., D. Befroy, S. Dufour, J. Dziura, C. Ariyan, D. L. Rothman, L. DiPietro, G. W. Cline, and G. I. Shulman. 2003. "Mitochondrial Dysfunction in the Elderly: Possible Role in Insulin Resistance." *Science* 300: 1140–1142.

Ravussin, E., M. E. Valencia, J. Esparza, P. H. Bennett, and L. O. Schulz. 1994. "Effects of a Traditional Lifestyle on Obesity in Pima Indians." *Diabetes Care* 17: 1067–1074.

Wang, Y., E. B. Rimm, M. J. Stampfer, W. C. Willett, and F. B. Hu. 2005. "Comparison of Abdominal Obesity and Overall Obesity in Predicting Risk of Type 2 Diabetes among Men." *American Journal of Clinical Nutrition* 81: 555–563.

13. Breaking the Insulin Cycle

Abu-Elheiga, L., M. M. Matzuk, K. A. H. Abo-Hashema, and S. J. Wakil. 2001. "Continuous Fatty Acid Oxidation and Reduced Fat Storage in Mice Lacking Acetyl-CoA Carboxylase 2." *Science* 291: 2613–2616.

Atkins, R. C. 2002. *Dr. Atkins' New Diet Revolution*. New York: M. Evans.

——— 2003. *Atkins for Life*. New York: St. Martin's.

Austin, M. A. 1999. "Epidemiology of Hypertriglyceridemia and Cardiovascular Disease." *American Journal of Cardiology* 83 (9B): 13F–16F.

Boden, G., K. Sargrad, C. Homko, M. Mozzoli, and T. P. Stein. 2005. "Effect of a Low-Carbohydrate Diet on Appetite, Blood Glucose Levels and Insulin Resistance in Obese Patients with Type 2 Diabetes." *Annals of Internal Medicine* 142: 403–411.

Brand-Miller, J. C., M. Thomas, V. Swan, Z. I. Ahmad, P. Petocz, and S. Colagiuri. 2003. "Physiological Validation of the Concept of Glycemic Load in Lean Young Adults." *Journal of Nutrition* 133: 2728–2732.

Bravata, D. M., L. Sanders, J. Huang, H. M. Krumholz, I. Olkin, C. D. Gardner, and D. M. Bravata. 2003. "Efficacy and Safety of Low-Carbohydrate Diets: A Systematic Review." *Journal of the American Medical Association* 289: 1837–1850.

Bray, G. A. 2003. "Low-Carbohydrate Diets and Realities of Weight Loss." *Journal of the American Medical Association* 289: 1853–1855.

Bray, G. A., S. J. Nielsen, and B. M. Popkin. 2004. "Consumption of High-Fructose Corn Syrup in Beverages May Play a Role in the Epidemic of Obesity." *American Journal of Clinical Nutrition* 79: 537–543.

Brehm, B. J., R. J. Seeley, S. R. Daniels, and D. A. D'Alessio. 2003. "A Randomized Trial Comparing a Very Low Carbohydrate Diet and a Calorie-Restricted Low Fat Diet on Body Weight and Cardiovascular Risk Factors in Healthy Women." *Journal of Clinical Endocrinology and Metabolism* 88:1617–1623.

Clarke, S. D. 2001. "Polyunsaturated Fatty Acid Regulation of Gene Transcription: A Molecular Mechanism to Improve the Metabolic Syndrome." *Journal of Nutrition* 131: 1129–1132.

Foster, G. D., H. R. Wyatt, J. O. Hill, B. G. McGuckin, C. Brill, B. S. Mohammed, P. O. Szapary, D. J. Rader, J. S. Edman, and S. Klein. 2003. "A Randomized Trial of a Low-Carbohydrate Diet for Obesity." *New England Journal of Medicine* 348: 2082–2090.

Foster-Powell, K., S. H. A. Holt, and J. C. Brand-Miller. 2002. "International Table of Glycemic Index and Glycemic Load Values: 2002." *American Journal of Nutrition* 76: 5–56.

Hudgins, L. C., M. Hellerstein, C. Seidman, R. Neese, J. Diakun, and J. Hirsch. 1996. "Human Fatty Acid Synthesis Is Stimulated by a Eucaloric Low Fat, High Carbohydrate Diet." *Journal of Clinical Investigation* 97: 2081–2091.

Hudgins, L. C., M. K. Hellerstein, C. E. Seidman, R. A. Neese, J. D. Tremaroli, and J. Hirsh. 2000. "Relationship between Carbohydrate-Induced Hypertriglyceridemia and Fatty Acid Synthesis in Lean and Obese Subjects." *Journal of Lipid Research* 41: 595–604.

Kersten, S., B. Desvergne, and W. Wahli. 2000. "Roles of PPARs in Health and Disease." *Nature* 405: 421–424.

Loftus, T. M., D. E. Jaworsky, G. L. Frehywot, C. A. Townsend, G. V. Ronnett, M. D. Lane, and F. P. Kuhajda. 2000. "Reduced Food Intake and Body Weight in Mice Treated with Fatty Acid Synthase Inhibitors." *Science* 288: 2379–2381.

Ludwig, D. S., K. E. Peterson, and S. L. Gortmaker. 2001. "Relationship between Consumption of Sugar-Sweetened Drinks and Childhood Obesity: A Prospective, Observational Analysis." *Lancet* 357: 505–508.

McDonald's Restaurants. 2004. "McDonald's Nutrition Facts for Popular Food Items." Accessed on October 5, 2004, at www.mcdonalds.com/app_controller.nutrition.categories.nutrition.index.html.

Neschen, S., I. Moore, W. Regittnig, C. L. Yu, Y. Wang, M. Pypaert, K. F. Petersen, and G. I. Shulman. 2002. "Contrasting Effects of Fish Oil and Safflower Oil on Hepatic Peroxisomal and Tissue Lipid Content." *American Journal of Physiology—Endocrinology and Metabolism* 282: E395–401.

Ornish, D. 2004. "Was Dr. Atkins Right?" *Journal of the American Dietetic Association* 104: 537–542.

Parks, E. J., and M. K. Hellerstein. 2000. "Carbohydrate-Induced Hypertriacylglycerolemia: Historical Perspective and Review of Biological Mechanisms." *American Journal of Clinical Nutrition* 71: 412–433.

Pescatore, F. 2004. *The Hamptons Diet.* Hoboken, NJ: John Wiley and Sons.

Pi-Sunyer, F. X. 2002. "Glycemic Index and Disease." *American Journal of Clinical Nutrition* 76 (suppl): 290S–298S.

Pizza Hut Restaurants. 2004. "Nutrition Information." Accessed on October 5, 2004, at www.pizzahut.com/menu/nutritioninfo.asp.

Reaven, G. M. 1988. "Role of Insulin Resistance in Human Disease." *Diabetes* 37: 1595–1607.

Reaven, G. M., T. K. Strom, and B. Fox. 2000. *Syndrome X: The Silent Killer, the New Heart Disease Risk.* New York: Simon and Schuster.

Samaha, F. F., N. Iqbal, P. Seshadri, K. L. Chicano, D. A. Daily, J. McGrory, T. Williams, M. Williams, E. J. Gracely, and L. Stern. 2003. "A Low-Carbohydrate as Compared with a Low-Fat Diet in Severe Obesity." *New England Journal of Medicine* 348: 2074–2081.

Sheard, N. F., N. G. Clark, J. C. Brand-Miller, M. J. Franz, F. X. Pi-Sunyer, E. Mayer-Davis, K. Kulkarni, and P. Geil. 2004. "Dietary Carbohydrate (Amount and Type) in the Prevention and Management of Diabetes." *Diabetes Care* 27: 2266–2271.

Smith, S. J., S. Cases, D. R. Jensen, H. C. Chen, E. Sande, B. Tow, D. A. Sanan, J. Raber, R. H. Eckel, and R. V. Farese. 2000. "Obesity Resistance and Multiple Mechanisms of Triglyceride Synthesis in Mice Lacking DGAT." *Nature Genetics* 25: 87–90.

Stern, L., N. Iqbal, P. Seshadri, K. L. Chicano, D. A. Daily, J. McGrory, M. Williams, E. J. Gracely, and F. F. Samaha. 2004. "The Effects of Low-Carbohydrate Versus Conventional Weight Loss Diets in Severely Obese Adults: One-Year Follow-up of a Randomized Trial." *Annals of Internal Medicine* 140: 778–785.

Steward, H. L., M. C. Bethea, S. S. Andrews, and L. A. Balart. 1995. *Sugar Busters! Cut Sugar to Trim Fat.* New Orleans: SugarBusters, LLC.

Taubes, G. 2001. "The Soft Science of Dietary Fat." *Science* 291: 2536–2545.

Yancy, W. S., M. K. Olsen, J. R. Guyton, R. P. Bakst, and E. C. Westman. 2004. "A Low-Carbohydrate, Ketogenic Diet Versus a Low-Fat Diet to Treat Obesity and Hyperlipidemia." *Annals of Internal Medicine* 140: 769–777.

Willett, W. C. 2001. *Eat, Drink, and Be Healthy.* New York: Simon & Schuster.

———— 2004. "Reduced-Carbohydrate Diets: No Roll in Weight Management?" *Annals of Internal Medicine* 140: 836–837.

Wood, P. A., D. M. Kurtz, K. B. Cox, L. R. Nyman, A. Elgavish, D. A. Hamm, B. A. Gower, and T. R. Nagy. 2003. "Role of Genetic Deficiency of Fatty Acid Oxidation in Metabolic Syndrome/Obesity." *Progress in Obesity Research* 9: 293–296.

14. Excercise to Burn Fat

Ainsworth, B. E., W. L. Haskell, A. S. Leon, D. R. Jacobs, Jr., H. J. Montoye, J. F. Sallis, and R. S. Paffenbarger, Jr. 1993. "Compendium of Physical Activities: Classification of Energy Costs of Human Physical Activities." *Medicine and Science in Sports and Exercise* 25: 71–80.

Goodpaster, B. H., J. He, S. Watkins, and D. E. Kelley. 2001. "Skeletal Muscle Lipid Content and Insulin Resistance: Evidence for a Paradox in Endurance-Trained Athletes." *Journal of Clinical Endocrinology and Metabolism* 86: 5755–5761.

Goodpaster, B. H., A. Katsiaras, and D. E. Kelley. 2003. "Enhanced Fat Oxidation through Physical Activity Is Associated with Improvements in Insulin Sensitivity in Obesity." *Diabetes* 52: 2191–2197.

Hallgren, P., L. Sjostrom, H. Hedlund, L. Lundell, and L. Olbe. 1989. "Influence of Age, Fat Cell Weight, and Obesity on O_2 Consumption of Human Adipose Tissue." *American Journal of Physiology—Endocrinology and Metabolism* 256: E467–E474.

He, J., B. H. Goodpaster, and D. E. Kelley. 2004. "Effects of Weight Loss and Physical Activity on Muscle Lipid Content and Droplet Size." *Obesity Research* 12: 761–769.

Hunter, G. R., J. P. McCarthy, and M. M. Bamman. 2004. "Effects of Resistance Training on Older Adults." *Sports Medicine* 34: 329–348.

Katzmarzyk, P. T., A. S. Leon, J. H. Wilmore, J. S. Skinner, D. C. Rao, T. Rankin, and C. Bouchard. 2003. "Targeting the Metabolic Syndrome with Exercise: Evidence from the HERITAGE Family Study." *Medicine and Science in Sports and Exercise* 35: 1703–1709.

Kearney, J. T. 2003. Lecture at University of Alabama at Birmingham, "Resting Metabolic Rate: Clinical Relevance, Technology of Assessment, Factors Affecting Variability, and the Contributions of Lean Muscle Mass." October 7. Available at http://138.26.176.127/CNRC/Seminars/JKearney/index.html.

Kelley, D. E. 2004. "Influence of Weight Loss and Physical Activity Interventions upon Muscle Lipid Content in Relation to Insulin Resistance." *Current Diabetes Reports* 4: 165–168.

Leon, A. S., S. E. Gaskill, T. Rice, J. Bergeron, J. Gagnon, D. C. Rao, J. S. Skinner, J. H.

Wilmore, and C. Bouchard. 2002. "Variability in the Response of HDL Cholesterol to Exercise Training in the HERITAGE Family Study." *International Journal of Sports Medicine* 23: 1–9.

Murray, R. K. 2000. "Muscle and the Cytoskeleton." In R. K. Murray, D. K. Granner, P. A. Mayes, and V. W. Rodwell, eds., *Harper's Biochemistry,* 715–736. New York: McGraw-Hill.

Nelson, K. M., R. L. Weinsier, C. L. Long, and Y. Schutz. 1992. "Prediction of Resting Energy Expenditure from Fat-Free Mass and Fat Mass." *American Journal of Clinical Nutrition* 56: 848–856.

Pruchnic, R., A. Katsiaras, J. He, C. Winters, D. E. Kelley, and B. H. Goodpaster. 2004. "Exercise Training Increases Intramyocellular Lipid and Oxidative Capacity in Older Adults." *American Journal of Physiology—Endocrinology and Metabolism* 287: E857–862.

Rauramaa, R., P. Halonen, S. B. Vaisanen, T. A. Lakka, A. Schmidt-Trucksass, A. Berg, I. M. Penttila, T. Rankinen, and C. Bouchard. 2004. "Effects of Aerobic Physical Exercise on Inflammation and Atherosclerosis in Men: The DNASCO Study." *Annals of Internal Medicine* 140: 1007–1014.

Speakman, J. R., and C. Selman. 2003. "Physical Activity and Resting Metabolic Rate." *Proceedings of the Nutrition Society* 62: 621–634.

Watkins, L. L., A. Sherwood, M. Feinglos, A. Hinderliter, M. Babyak, E. Gullette, R. Waugh, and J. A. Blumenthal. 2003. "Effects of Exercise and Weight Loss on Cardiac Risk Factors Associated with Syndrome X." *Archives of Internal Medicine* 163: 1889–1895.

15. Lipid-Lowering Drugs

Benecol Products. 2004. "Frequently Asked Questions." Accessed on October 14, 2004, at www.benecol.com/contactus/index.jhtml?id=benecol/contactus/faq_main.inc.

Bloch, K. 1965. "The Biological Synthesis of Cholesterol." *Science* 15: 19–28.

Endo, A. 1992. "The Discovery and Development of HMG-CoA Reductase Inhibitors." *Journal of Lipid Research* 33: 1569–1582.

General Accounting Office. 2002. "Prescription Drugs—FDA Oversight of Direct-to-Consumer Advertising Has Limitations." Washington, DC: U.S. General Accounting Office, Report to Congressional Requestors GAE-03-177. Accessed at www.gao.gov/new.items/d03177.pdf.

Gotto, A. M. 1999. *Contemporary Diagnosis and Management of Lipid Disorders.* Newtown, PA: Handbooks in Healthcare.

Goetzman, E.S, L. Tian, T. R. Nagy, B. A. Gower, T. R. Schoeb, A. Elgavish, E. P. Acosta, M. S. Saag, and P. A. Wood. 2003. "HIV Protease Inhibitor Ritonavir Induces Lipoatrophy in Male Mice." *AIDS Research and Human Retroviruses* 19: 1141–1150.

Goldberg, I. J., C. F. Semenkovich, and H. N. Ginsberg. 2000. "Diabetes Mellitus and

Vascular Risk." In P. W. F. Wilson, ed., *Atlas of Atherosclerosis*, 193–212. Philadelphia: Current Medicine.

Henkin, Y., K. C. Johnson, and J. P. Segrest. 1990. "Rechallenge with Crystalline Niacin after Drug-Induced Hepatitis from Sustained-Release Niacin." *Journal of the American Medical Association* 264: 241–243.

Hunninghake, D. B., and E. A. Stein. 2000. "Lipid-Lowering Drugs." In P. W. F. Wilson, ed., *Atlas of Atherosclerosis*, 156–177. Philadelphia: Current Medicine.

Jaret, P. 2001. "Ten Ways to Improve Patient Compliance." *Hippocrates* February/March: 22–28.

Junod, S. W. 2003. "Sugar: A Cautionary Tale." Food and Drug Law Institute *Update*, July–August. Accessed at www.fda.gov/oc/history/makinghistory/sugar.html.

Lebovitz, H. E. 1999. "Effects of Oral Antihyperglycemic Agents in Modifying Macrovascular Risk Factors in Type 2 Diabetes." *Diabetes Care* 22 [Suppl. 3]: C41–44.

Levy, R. I., A. J. Troendle, and J. M. Fattu. 1993. "A Quarter Century of Drug Treatment of Dyslipoproteinemia, with a Focus on the New HMG-CoA Reductase Inhibitor Fluvastatin." *Circulation* 87 [Suppl. III]: III-45–53.

Miettinen, T. A., P. Puska, H. Gylling, H. Vanhanen, and E. Vartiainen. 1995. "Reduction of Serum Cholesterol with Sitostanol-Ester Margarine in a Mildly Hypercholesterolemic Population." *New England Journal of Medicine* 333: 1308–1312.

Rodenburg, J., M. Vissers, A. Wiegman, M. Trip, H. Bakker, and J. J. Kastelein. 2004. "Familial Hypercholesterolemia in Children." *Current Opinion in Lipidology* 15: 405–411.

Schoonjans, K., B. Staels, and J. Auwerx. 1996. "Role of Peroxisome Proliferator-Activated Receptor (PPAR) in Mediating the Effects of Fibrates and Fatty Acids on Gene Expression." *Journal of Lipid Research* 37: 907–925.

Sotos, J. G. 2003. "Taft and Pickwick: Sleep Apnea in the White House." *CHEST* 124: 1133–1142.

Take Control Products. 2004. "Get to Know Take Control [link to FAQs]." Accessed on October 14, 2004, at *www.takecontrol.com/getknow/default.htm*.

Witztum, J. L. 1996. "Drugs Used in the Treatment of Hyperlipoproteinemias." In J. G. Hardman, L. E. Limbird, P. B. Molinoff, and R. W. Ruddon, eds., *The Pharmacological Basis of Therapeutics*, 875–897. New York: McGraw-Hill.

Zhou, G., R. Myers, Y. Li, Y. Chen, X. Shen, J. Fenyk-Melody, M. Wu, J. Ventre, T. Doebber, N. Fujii, N. Musi, M. F. Hirshman, L. J. Goodyear, and D. E. Moller. 2001. "Role of AMP-Activated Protein Kinase in Mechanism of Metformin Action." *Journal of Clinical Investigation* 108: 1167–1174.

16. Practical Lessons for Making Good Decisions

Critser, G. 2003. *Fat Land.* Boston: Houghton Mifflin.

Esposito, K., R. Marfella, M. Ciotola, C. Di Palo, F. Giugliano, G. Giugliano, M.

D'Armiento, F. D'Andrea, and D. Giugliano. 2004. "Effect of a Mediterranean-Style Diet on Endothelial Dysfunction and Markers of Vascular Inflammation in the Metabolic Syndrome." *Journal of the American Medical Association* 292: 1440–1446.

Friedman, J. M. 2003. "A War on Obesity, Not the Obese." *Science* 299: 856–858.

Knoops, K. T. B., L. C. P. G. de Groot, D. Kromhout, A.-E. Perrin, O. Moreiras-Varela, A. Menotti, and W. A. van Staveren. 2004. "Mediterranean Diet, Lifestyle Factors, and 10-Year Mortality in Elderly European Men and Women." *Journal of the American Medical Association* 292: 1433–1439.

Kolata, G. 2004. "The Fat Epidemic: He Says It's an Illusion." *New York Times*, June 8.

Rimm, E. B., and M. J. Stampfer. 2004. "Diet, Lifestyle, and Longevity—The Next Steps?" *Journal of the American Medical Association* 292: 1490–1492.

Schlosser, E. 2001. *Fast Food Nation*. Boston: Houghton Mifflin.

Shell, E. R. 2002. *The Hungry Gene*. New York: Grove Press.

17. Nutrient Labeling

Bender, M. M., J. J. Rader, and F. D. McClure. 1998. *Guidance for Industry: FDA Nutrition Labeling Manual—A Guide for Developing and Using Data Bases*. Washington, DC: U.S. Food and Drug Administration. Accessed at www.cfsan.fda.gov/~dms/nutrguid.html; updated January 11, 2005.

Food and Drug Administration (FDA). 1994. "A Food Labeling Guide—Appendix A—Definitions of Nutrient Content Claims." Washington, DC: U.S. Food and Drug Administration. Accessed at www.cfsan.fda.gov/~dms/flg-6a.html; updated October 2004.

——— 1999. "The Food Label." Washington, DC: U.S. Food and Drug Administration. Accessed at www.cfsan.fda.gov/~dms/fdnewlab.html; updated July 9, 2003.

Hu, F. B., and W. C. Willett. 2002. "Optimal Diets for Prevention of Coronary Heart Disease." *Journal of the American Medical Association* 288: 2569–2578.

Kurtzweil, P. 1993. "Good Reading for Good Eating." *FDA Consumer*, May. Accessed at www.cfsan.fda.gov/~dms/fdlabel2.html#milestone.

18. Alternative Medicine and Fad Diets

Anderson, R. A., C. L. Broadhurst, M. M. Polansky, W. F. Schmidt, A. Khan, V. P. Flanagan, N. W. Schoene, and D. J. Graves. 2004. "Isolation and Characterization of Polyphenol Type-A Polymers from Cinnamon with Insulin-like Biological Activity." *Journal of Agricultural and Food Chemistry* 52: 65–70.

Gray, A. M, P. R. Flatt. 1997. "Pancreatic and Extra-Pancreatic Effects of the Traditional Anti-Diabetic Plant, *Medicago sativa* (Lucerne)." *British Medical Journal* 78: 325–334.

Khan, A., M. Safdar, M. H. A. Khan, K. N. Khattak, and R. A. Anderson. 2003. "Cinnamon Improves Glucose and Lipids in People with Type 2 Diabetes." *Diabetes Care* 26: 3215–3218.

19. Media Coverage of Health Research

Alberts, D. S., M. E. Martinez, D. J. Roe, J. M. Guillen-Rodriguez, J. R. Marshall, J. B. Van Leeuwen, M. E. Reid, C. Ritenbaugh, P. A. Vargas, A. B. Bhattacharyya, D. L. Earnest, R. E. Sampliner, and the Phoenix Colon Cancer Prevention Physician's Network. 2000. "Lack of Effect of a High–Fiber Cereal Supplement on the Recurrence of Colorectal Adenomas." *New England Journal of Medicine* 342: 1156–1162.

Burkitt, D. P. 1971. "Epidemiology of Cancer of the Colon and Rectum." *Cancer* 28: 3–13.

National Center for Health Statistics (NCHS). 2005. "Life Expectancy." Accessed at http://www.cdc.gov/nchs/data/hus/hus04trend.pdf#027; updated May 30, 2005.

Reaven, G., T. K. Strom, and B. Fox. 2000. *Syndrome X: The Silent Killer, the New Heart Disease Risk.* New York: Simon and Schuster.

Schatzkin, A., E. Lanza, D. Corle, P. Lance, F. Iber, B. Caan, M. Shike, J. Weissfeld, R. Burt, M. R. Cooper, J. W. Kikendall, J. Cahill, and the Polyp Prevention Trial Study Group. 2000. "Lack of Effect of a Low-Fat, High-Fiber Diet on the Recurrence of Colorectal Adenomas." *New England Journal of Medicine* 342: 1149–1155.

Willett, W. C. 2001. *Eat, Drink, and Be Healthy.* New York: Simon and Schuster.

Further Reading

Mayes, P. A. 2000. "Biosynthesis of Fatty Acids." In R. K. Murray, D. K. Granner, P. A. Mayes, and V. W. Rodwell, eds., *Harper's Biochemistry,* 230–237. New York: McGraw-Hill.

Mayes, P. A. 2000. "Cholesterol Synthesis, Transport and Excretion." In R. K. Murray, D. K. Granner, P. A. Mayes, and V. W. Rodwell, eds., *Harper's Biochemistry,* 285–297. New York: McGraw-Hill.

Mayes, P. A. 2000. "Lipids of Physiological Significance." In R. K. Murray, D. K. Granner, P. A. Mayes, and V. W. Rodwell, eds., *Harper's Biochemistry,* 160–171. New York: McGraw-Hill.

Mayes, P. A. 2000. "Oxidation of Fatty Acids: Ketogenesis." In R. K. Murray, D. K. Granner, P. A. Mayes, and V. W. Rodwell, eds., *Harper's Biochemistry,* 238–249. New York: McGraw-Hill.

Index